CANCER ETIOLOGY, DIAGNOSIS AND TREATMENTS

ROLE OF PROSTATE-SPECIFIC ANTIGEN (PSA) IN PATHOLOGICAL ANGIOGENESIS AND PROSTATE TUMOR GROWTH

Cancer Etiology, Diagnosis and Treatments

Additional books in this series can be found on Nova's website under the Series tab.

Additional E-books in this series can be found on Nova's website under the E-book tab.

CANCER ETIOLOGY, DIAGNOSIS AND TREATMENTS

ROLE OF PROSTATE-SPECIFIC ANTIGEN (PSA) IN PATHOLOGICAL ANGIOGENESIS AND PROSTATE TUMOR GROWTH

RAVIKUMAR AALINKEEL
STANLEY A. SCHWARTZ
B. BINDUKUMAR
GARY J. SMITH
AND
KAILASH C. CHADHA

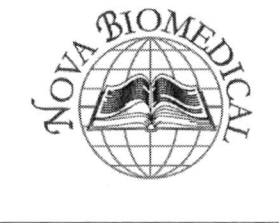

Nova Biomedical Books
New York

Copyright © 2012 by Nova Science Publishers, Inc.

All rights reserved. No part of this book may be reproduced, stored in a retrieval system or transmitted in any form or by any means: electronic, electrostatic, magnetic, tape, mechanical photocopying, recording or otherwise without the written permission of the Publisher.

For permission to use material from this book please contact us:
Telephone 631-231-7269; Fax 631-231-8175
Web Site: http://www.novapublishers.com

NOTICE TO THE READER

The Publisher has taken reasonable care in the preparation of this book, but makes no expressed or implied warranty of any kind and assumes no responsibility for any errors or omissions. No liability is assumed for incidental or consequential damages in connection with or arising out of information contained in this book. The Publisher shall not be liable for any special, consequential, or exemplary damages resulting, in whole or in part, from the readers' use of, or reliance upon, this material. Any parts of this book based on government reports are so indicated and copyright is claimed for those parts to the extent applicable to compilations of such works.

Independent verification should be sought for any data, advice or recommendations contained in this book. In addition, no responsibility is assumed by the publisher for any injury and/or damage to persons or property arising from any methods, products, instructions, ideas or otherwise contained in this publication.

This publication is designed to provide accurate and authoritative information with regard to the subject matter covered herein. It is sold with the clear understanding that the Publisher is not engaged in rendering legal or any other professional services. If legal or any other expert assistance is required, the services of a competent person should be sought. FROM A DECLARATION OF PARTICIPANTS JOINTLY ADOPTED BY A COMMITTEE OF THE AMERICAN BAR ASSOCIATION AND A COMMITTEE OF PUBLISHERS.

Additional color graphics may be available in the e-book version of this book.

Library of Congress Cataloging-in-Publication Data

ISBN: 978-1-61122-975-2

Published by Nova Science Publishers, Inc. † New York

Contents

Preface		vii
Chapter I	Prostate Cancer Statistics	1
Chapter II	Biology of PSA and Regulation by Androgen	3
Chapter III	PSA in Blood	5
Chapter IV	PSA Screening and Early Detection of CaP	7
Chapter V	Angiogenic Growth Factors and Cytokines Associated with CaP Growth, Metastasis and Invasion	9
Chapter VI	Role of PSA in CaP Angiogenesis	17
Chapter VII	Isolation and Characterization of Human PSA for Evaluation of the Physiological Role of PSA in Angiogenesis	19
Chapter VIII	Purification and Characterization of f-PSA from Seminal Plasma	23
Chapter IX	Role of f-PSA in Angiogenesis and Prostate Tumor Growth: Gene Expression Profile	27
Chapter X	Role of PSA in Angiogenesis by Endothelial Cells *In Vitro*	31

Chapter XI	Effect of Treatment of CaP Cells (PC-3M) with f-PSA on the Differential Expression of Proteins	33
Conclusion		41
Acknowledgements		47
References		49
Index		65

Preface

Prostate specific antigen (PSA) is a serine protease present in an enzymatically inactive form in human serum at a concentration of nanograms/ml; serum PSA (S-PSA) is used widely as a surrogate marker in the diagnosis and management of prostate cancer (CaP). However, the vast majority of PSA produced in the prostate is secreted as active enzyme into the seminal fluid (SF-PSA: milligram/ml) or is sequestered within the prostate tissue microenvironment (T-PSA) µg/gm of tissue). Furthermore, PSA is present in multiple androgen receptor (AR) expressing human tissues and fluids, including parotid tissue, endometrium, normal breast tissue, breast milk and female serum, and human cancers, including parotid tumors, breast carcinoma, renal cell carcinoma, and ovarian cancer. The enzymatically active PSA sequestered in prostate tissue (T-PSA) potentially represents the pool most critical to the pathogenesis of prostate cancer, however, the role of T-PSA in the onset, progression, and metastasis is not well understood. PSA levels within the tissue microenvironment are reduced in prostate cancer compared to benign prostate, and can fall to undetectable levels in advanced cancer. T- PSA levels correlate with prognosis in both prostate cancer and breast cancer; the higher the T-PSA level, the better the prognosis. We have shown that incubation of PC-3M human prostate cancer cells with purified PSA *in vitro* results in down-regulation of expression of genes/proteins associated with prostate cancer progression, including multiple genes associated with angiogenesis, and administration of purified PSA to the tumor microenvironment of PC-3M xenografts engrafted to immuno-compromised hosts resulted in inhibition of tumor growth. Furthermore, we have shown that purified PSA inhibited significantly, in a dose dependent manner, the migration, chemotaxis and attachment functions of Human Umbilical Vein

Endothelial cells (HUVEC) cells required for tube formation in the *in vitro* in the Matrigel 'angiogenesis assay". Significantly, both enzymatically active and inactive forms of PSA had anti-angiogenic activity *in vitro* Matrigel assay suggesting that biological function of PSA may be mediated through factors other than just enzymatic function. Consequently, re-introduction of PSA into the prostate (or possibly breast) tissue microenvironment could provide a non-immunogenic, tissue-specific, mechanistically-based therapy to block tumor angiogenesis.

Chapter I

Prostate Cancer Statistics

Prostate cancer (CaP) is the most frequently diagnosed, non-cutaneous malignancy of men in the industrialized world. CaP diagnosis, which is increasing globally, varies among countries, with the US, Canada, Sweden, Australia, and France having the highest rates [1]. In 2005 (the most recent year for which data are available), 185,895 new cases of CaP were diagnosed in the US, and 28,905 men died from this cancer. The American Cancer Society estimated that in 2009 there would be 191,532 new cases of CaP in the US, which will comprise 25% of all male cancers diagnosed, with 26,328 estimated deaths. The incidence and mortality of CaP in the US is significantly higher in African-American men compared to other ethnic and racial groups [2-4]. With ~200,000 new cases of CaP being diagnosed every year in the US as a consequence of wide-spread serum PSA-based screening, an increasing proportion of newly diagnosed men present with low-grade, low-stage disease compared to the pre-PSA era. This phenomenon of "stage migration" has spurred considerable investigation into the biology and mechanistic role of PSA in CaP. This review summarizes the biology, biochemistry and physiology of PSA with relevance to CaP biology and angiogenesis.

Chapter II

Biology of PSA and Regulation by Androgen

PSA is an androgen-regulated serine protease of the tissue kallikrein (KLK) family that possesses a chymotrypsin-like activity [5]. PSA (KLK3) is produced in benign prostate and benign prostatic hyperplasia (BPH) by the glandular or secretory epithelial cells and in CaP by prostate cancer epithelial cells of all grades and stages [6,7]. PSA is modified post-translationally in the Golgi and secreted into seminal fluid, in which PSA concentrations range from ~0.3 to 3 mg/ml (10–100 µM) [8]. The majority of PSA in seminal plasma is an active serine protease with chymotrypsin-like activity responsible for proteolysis of the gel proteins of seminal fluid (for example, semenogelin I & II [9] enhancing sperm mobility by liquefying seminal fluid [9,10]. However, PSA gene expression also is detectable in parotid gland, endometrium [11], normal breast tissue [12], breast milk [13], female serum [12], breast cancer [14,15], adrenal neoplasms [16], renal cell carcinoma [16], and ovarian cancer [17].

In humans, the genes for all 15 glandular KLK are clustered in a locus that spans approximately 280 kb of chromosome 19q133–4 [18]. Transcription of PSA is regulated by androgens through androgen receptor (AR) mediated transactivation conferred by androgen response elements in the promoter of the PSA/KLK3 gene. The closest paralogue of KLK3, KLK2 (encoding human kallikrein 2 (hK2)) is also androgen-regulated through androgen response elements (AREs). Although 11 of the 15 human kallikrein genes appear to be evolutionarily conserved, the KLK3 and KLK2 genes underwent major changes during mammalian evolution [19]. The genomes of mice and rats do not contain functional alleles of KLK2 or KLK3, but instead contain 1–10 pseudo-gene copies of a KLK2 and/or KLK3 progenitor [19]. Functional KLK3 genes are found only in primates, and functional KLK2 genes are limited to primates and dogs [19]. This is notable because humans, primates and dogs are the few species known to spontaneously develop BPH and prostate cancer. The canine KLK2 promoter contains AREs, whereas, the rodent pseudo-genes lack these elements [18]. AR is the primary regulator of PSA expression. AR bound to dihydrotestosterone (DHT), the most potent ligand for wild-type AR, induces PSA expression through three ARE-containing enhancer elements located in the proximal 6 kb of the PSA promoter [20,21]. The androgen-independent prostate cancer cell line PC-3, which does not express either AR or PSA, demonstrated androgen-stimulation of PSA production only after transfection of AR, validating the importance of AR activity for PSA expression [22]. In addition to androgen, PSA expression was induced by glucocorticoids in T47D breast cancer cells[23] and in LNCaP cells transfected with the glucocorticoid receptor [24]. Progestins stimulated PSA expression at low concentrations (10^{-11} to 10^{-10} M) in breast cancer cell lines [23,25], and oral contraceptives that contained progestin induced PSA expression in breast tissue [26]. Recently, a novel transcription factor, GAGATA binding protein, was identified and found to affect androgen-mediated expression of PSA through binding to an alternative enhancer site (GAGATA) in the PSA promoter [27]. Two E twenty-six (Ets) family transcription factors, epithelium-specific Ets factor 2 (ESE2) and prostate-derived Ets factor (PDEF), were reported to induce transcription of a PSA reporter gene in the AR-negative cell line CV-1 [28,29]. PDEF is highly expressed in prostate and weakly expressed in the ovary [29]. Although PDEF is capable of inducing PSA expression in the absence of AR, PDEF can hetero-dimerize with AR to enhance AR-induced transcription [29]. ESE2 is expressed weakly in the normal prostate, and it is not known whether this transcription factor directly interacts with AR [28]. The ability of Ets transcription factors to regulate PSA expression in prostate cancer remains to be determined. A small percentage of cells in local prostate tumors have been found to express PSA but lack detectable AR expression by immuno-histochemistry [30]. It is possible that PSA expression in these cells is regulated by an Ets transcription factor. As discussed above, the majority of prostate tumors express AR, and therefore the significance of AR-independent PSA expression is unclear.

Chapter III

PSA in Blood

The normal prostate architecture separates the secretory or luminal epithelial cells from the microvasculature of the relatively avascular prostate tissue microenvironment, such that only a minute proportion of PSA leaks into the circulation. PSA is present in the serum (S-PSA) of post-pubertal males at nanogram quantities, with >90% of S-PSA present as complexes with protease inhibitors, including α_2-macroglobulin and α_1-anti-chymotrypsin (ACT). The protease inhibitors are present at a 10^5-fold excess, and inactivate any catalytic PSA by forming stable covalent complexes [31,32]. Consequently, S-PSA manifests little or no catalytic activity [31,33]. However, small amounts of S-PSA exist as a free pro-protein or mature protein that may be intact or enzymatically nicked. The multiple forms of S-PSA, and the implications for prostate cancer, will be discussed further below. PSA levels in the blood span a 10^5-fold range, from <0.1 to 10^4 ng/ml, with levels above 10^2 ng/ml found almost exclusively in men with advanced prostate cancer. PSA levels in blood also are influenced by other prostate disease conditions, such as BPH and prostatitis, and by age, body mass index and race. It has been observed that after age 50, the median PSA level increases, most probably as a result of the increasing occurrence of benign prostate diseases with age: BPH, for example, is found in only a few percent of 40 year olds but in a quarter of 60 year olds [34]. Because of this rise in PSA, age-specific reference ranges have been proposed as a means of increasing the sensitivity of detection in younger men and the specificity in older men [35,36]. Age-specific ranges have, however, been criticized, mainly for missing clinically significant cancers in older men [37], and have not become uniformly accepted. PSA secreted into seminal fluid, in contrast, is present at concentrations of 0.2-3.0 mg/mL, a level six orders of magnitude higher than in serum, with >90% of the PSA in seminal fluid (SF-PSA) present as uncomplexed and enzymatically active protein [38,39]. Finally, a third, and largely uncharacterized, pool of PSA is sequestered within the prostate tissue microenvironment (T-PSA). T-PSA is present in microgram quantities, a level three orders of magnitude greater than S-PSA, and in contrast to S-PSA essentially all T-PSA is enzymatically active [40]. Importantly, T-PSA levels correlate with the level of expression of PSA by the prostate epithelial/cancer epithelial cells, and with the physiological state of the prostate gland: T-PSA levels are highest in benign prostate tissue, and decrease progressively with increasing grade and stage of prostate cancer [41,42]. Whether variations in PSA level between individuals are influenced by genetics is an area of active research, but, as yet, definitive data is lacking. The increased blood levels of PSA in men with cancer cannot be explained by increased PSA expression; during the development and progression of prostate cancer, PSA expression may actually decrease in cancer cells [43]. Downregulation of PSA expression in both prostate [40,44] and breast cancer tissue [45] has been correlated with more aggressive cancers and poorer prognosis [46]. Although there are no experimental data on the mechanisms of increased release, PSA in serum is believed to result from the disruption of prostate architecture in prostate tumors, such as loss of the basement membrane with disruption of the basal cell layer, ductal lumen architecture and epithelial cell polarity. Consequently, the inverse relationship where S-PSA levels increase with progression of prostate cancer, even though the cancer cells are producing significantly lower levels of PSA, highlights the lack of understanding of the role of PSA in prostate cancer progression. The enhanced levels of circulating PSA in prostate cancer that correlate with disease-free survival rate and distant metastasis-free survival rate are of unknown significance to disease progression [42,46,47]. Significantly, T-PSA may represent a superior prognostic marker compared to serum PSA because T-PSA levels are not dependent upon the mechanism(s) of transport/clearance of T-PSA into the blood. In contrast, T-PSA levels correlate to increased grade, and tumor stage, with highly malignant tumors having low levels of PSA m-RNA and T-PSA. [42,43,48].

Chapter IV

PSA Screening and Early Detection of CaP

In the United States, PSA was approved by the Food and Drug Administration as a marker to monitor patients treated for prostate cancer in 1986, and as a diagnostic marker in 1994. As PSA-based screening became widespread in the United States, it led to an apparent increased incidence of prostate cancer and to stage migration, resulting in a decreased proportion of metastatic or locally advanced cancers at diagnosis [49]. There is unquestionable evidence that prostate cancer risk varies with the levels of PSA circulating in the blood [50-53]. However, assessing the value of the serum PSA test involves several difficulties. As noted above, serum PSA levels vary with age and various other factors, and this hampers comparison between studies [34-37]. In addition, most studies of PSA testing are subject to verification bias, which is described in more detail below. In the context of detecting prostate cancer, an increased PSA level prompts a recommendation that the man undergo prostate biopsy, with PSA of > 4 ng/ml being the traditional threshold level. In three studies of large cohorts without extensive prior screening, men with PSA above this threshold had cancer detection rates of 27–44% [54-56]. The specificity and sensitivity of PSA testing have been harder to determine, because the prostate cancer status of men with low PSA values is seldom verified by biopsy. The Prostate Cancer Prevention Trial (PCPT), however, is unique in requesting that all participants undergo biopsy. Among 5,112 men in the placebo arm of this trial, a PSA level >4 ng/ml had specificity of 93% and sensitivity of 24% [57]. The threshold of PSA $\geq$4 ng/ml is frequently criticized, on the one hand for being too lax and on the other for being too strict. Numerous studies have reported that prostate cancer is not rare in men with PSA values <4 ng/ml. For example, among men with a median age of 72 years in the placebo arm of the PCPT, prostate cancer was detected by biopsy in 6.6% of men with PSA <0.5 ng/ml and in 27% of men with PSA 3.1–4 ng/ml [58]. Similarly, a large European study reported a cumulative prostate cancer detection rate of 21–25% for men with PSA of 2.0–2.99 ng/ml, and 33% at PSA 3.0–3.99 ng/ml [50]. Results from the PCPT in particular, however, demonstrate that use of lower PSA thresholds increases sensitivity at the expense of specificity, and that no cut-point achieves both high sensitivity and high specificity [59]. There is increasing appreciation, although no consensus, that a single PSA cut-point for recommending prostate biopsy might be inappropriate. First, no single cut-point distinguishes men into two homogenous groups of high and low cancer risk [51-53]. Second, the risk at which men would opt for biopsy is strongly influenced by personal preference, age, heredity, race and presence of concurrent disease. Accordingly, there has been a move towards calculating a percentage probability of prostate cancer based on the PSA level and on additional predictors of cancer risk, then presenting this probability to the patient as part of shared decision on biopsy. An online calculator, developed by the PCPT investigators, uses PSA and other risk factors to provide a continuous estimate of cancer risk, rather than a binary positive or negative test result [60].

Chapter V

Angiogenic Growth Factors and Cytokines Associated with CaP Growth, Metastasis and Invasion

Angiogenesis is a complex process that stimulates new blood vessels from existing vasculature [61-63]. Under normal conditions, this tightly regulated process occurs only during embryonic development, during the female reproductive cycle, and during wound healing. In contrast, in several pathological conditions, such as cancer, rheumatoid arthritis, atherosclerosis and diabetic retinopathy, angiogenesis becomes persistent due to an imbalance in the interplay between positive and negative regulatory signals that control the process [64,65]. Furthermore, not only is the pathogenesis of the primary cancer dependent on angiogenesis, but the establishment of metastases also is highly dependent on angiogenesis at the distant site [61,65-70]. Tumor angiogenesis, the formation of new blood vessels by endothelial cell proliferation, motility of endothelial cells through the extra-cellular matrix toward angiogenic stimuli, and capillary differentiation [66], is a feature of aggressive tumors and may be highly dysregulated by a perturbation of the dynamic interplay between stimulatory and inhibitory signals [64,71]. A number of regulatory factors that participate in the angiogenic process, including proliferative and migratory signaling molecules and their receptors, proteases, integrins and other adhesion molecules have been identified [66], including stimulatory factors such as vascular endothelial growth factor (VEGF), transforming growth factor (TGF)-β, tumor necrosis factor (TNF)-α, platelet derived growth factor (PDGF), and interleukin (IL)-8 [69,70], and inhibitory factors, including specific cytokines, interferons (IFNs), IL-12 and matrix glycoproteins [61,72]. Among the pro-angiogenic factors, the angiogenesis activator, VEGF [73], has been reported to be produced by CaP cells at far greater levels than by cells from BPH or normal prostate epithelial [74]. VEGF has been reported also to be expressed at low levels by stromal cells of the normal prostate [75]. Studies focused on the mechanistic effects of increased VEGF expression have confirmed that VEGF over-expression was directly responsible for enhanced tumorigenicity by human CaP cells [76,77]. Further, the role of VEGF in CaP progression has been confirmed using anti-VEGF antibodies for treatment [78,79]. In these studies treatment with anti-VEGF antibody suppressed angiogenesis, tumor growth, and metastasis, even in well-established tumors. Of the other pro-angiogenic factors, members of the chemokine family, specifically IL-8, contributed to both growth and progression of different types of human cancer. Chemokines are divided into two major subfamilies (CC and CXC) based on the position of their NH_2-terminal cysteine residues, that bind to seven transmembrane domain G-protein–coupled receptors, with two major subfamilies designated CCR and CXCR. IL-8 is a member of the CXC chemokine family; it is chemotactic for and activates leukocytes. IL-8 also has mitogenic and , angiogenic properties in a wide variety of human solid tumors including malignant melanoma; non–small cell lung cancer; malignant mesothelioma; head and neck squamous carcinoma; cervical and endometrial carcinoma; epithelial ovarian carcinoma; gastric, pancreatic, and colorectal carcinoma; hepatocellular carcinoma; androgen-independent prostate adenocarcinoma; renal cell carcinoma; breast cancer; and Kaposi's sarcoma [80-92]. IL-8 is secreted by a variety of stromal cells, *e.g.*, endothelial cells and fibroblasts, and tumor cells, *e.g.*, melanoma, prostate, and endometrial tumor cells. IL-8 binds with high specificity to CXCR-1, and with less specificity to CXCR-2 [93]. Both receptors are expressed on stromal cells and tumor cells [94]. The exact mechanisms by which IL-8 promotes tumor growth remains to be determined, although some studies suggest an autocrine role of IL-8 in modulating survival and proliferation of tumor cells [95]. Additionally, autocrine and/or paracrine modulation of tumor cells to further enhance an IL-8-mediated chemo-resistant phenotype also has been proposed [96]. Clinical studies have shown mRNA transcripts of IL-8 in normal tissues, as well as in both stromal and tumor cells of neoplastic tissues [81]. However the same study did not show any correlation between the expression of IL-8 mRNA and clinico-pathological variables, such as tumor grade, patient age, or nodal status; however, significantly higher levels of expression of IL-8 were measured in neoplastic tissues compared with normal tissues [81]. Furthermore, increased IL-8 expression in metastasis-prone cell lines has been observed and is believed to be caused by an atypical epigenetic mechanism whereby upstream cytosine and guanine separated by a phosphate (CpG) methylation, rather than promoter methylation [97]. Additionally, pre-clinical studies have confirmed that the expression of IL-8 in CaP cells correlated with angiogenesis, tumorigenicity and metastasis of experimental prostate cancer in athymic nude mice [83,98]. These *in vivo* observations are further supported by *in vitro* experiments that demonstrated IL-8 increased the invasiveness of prostate cancer cells by regulating matrix metalloproteinase synthesis and secretion [83,98,99], and was associated with progression of the LNCaP prostate cancer cell line toward androgen-independent growth [100]. Clinical studies have reported increased expression of IL-8 in the serum of prostate cancer patients in comparison with normal subjects or patients with BPH [101]. Furthermore, genetic studies have reported that the frequency of a specific polymorphism in the IL-8 gene promoter that results in elevated IL-8 expression is more prevalent in patients with metastatic prostate cancer compared with normal controls [102]. In addition to acting upon cancer cells, extracellular secretion of IL-8 from CaP cells modulated the activity of other cell types within the tumor microenvironment. For example, the pro-angiogenic activity of IL-8 can act upon the endothelial compartment of the tumor to induce neo-vascularization [103]. Secondly, the chemotactic activity of IL-8 has a profound effect in recruiting neutrophils and macrophages to the tumor site and inducing their tumor-promoting activity [104]. Additionally, cancer cell derived IL-8 has been associated with the potentiation of bone metastasis in CaP. IL-8 also has been shown to promote osteoclastogenesis and bone resorption through a Receptor Activator for Nuclear Factor κB Ligand (RANKL) independent mechanism that has not been characterized [105]. Our own study of prostate cancer cells demonstrated elevated expression and secretion of IL-8, suggesting that CaP cells are subject to continuous autocrine/paracrine IL-8 stimulation, the magnitude of which was greatest in the most aggressive prostate cancer cell line, PC-3 [73]. To investigate this correlation, we used the highly aggressive prostate cancer cell lines, PC-3 and PC-3M, to examine the role of IL-8 and IL-8 receptors in the aggressive phenotype. Consistent with our earlier report of increased IL-8 secretion by PC-3 cells [73], we confirmed this finding and extended the observation to PC-3M cells, and a derivative of PC-3M cells, PC3-MM2, characterized to be much more aggressive than PC-3 cells, to demonstrate the highly aggressive cells produced progressively greater levels of secretion of IL-8 compared to the parental cells. We quantitated IL-8 by ELISA in culture supernates of PC-3M and PC-3MM2 and observed significantly higher levels of IL-8 in these two cell lines compared to the parental, PC-3 cells (unpublished data). As the IL-8 signal is mediated in these cells through their corresponding IL-8 receptors, we determined the expression of the IL-8 receptors, CXCR1 and CXCR2, in PC-3 and PC-3M cells, and found significantly elevated levels of expression as determined by immunofluorence (data not shown). Abundant CXCR1 protein, but low levels of CXCR2 protein, were detected on the surface of the PC-3 and PC-3M cells (data not shown). In contrast, negligible expression of either CXCR1 or CXCR2 was detected by flow cytometry on the surface of LNCaP cells which do not manifest an aggressive phenotype . Serum from normal healthy controls (n= 25), patients with BPH (n= 32), and prostate cancer patients (n= 25) were analyzed for the presence of IL-8 and PSA using commercially available reagents (Figure 1 unpublished data). Serum levels of IL-8 are significantly higher in prostate cancer patients as compared to control and BPH patients. However, no significant differences were seen between controls and BPH sera. PSA serum levels were higher, both in BPH and prostate cancer patients compared to controls. This suggests that IL-8 measurements can facilitate the distinction between BPH and prostate cancer patients; which is not possible based on PSA measurements alone (Figure 1 unpublished data).

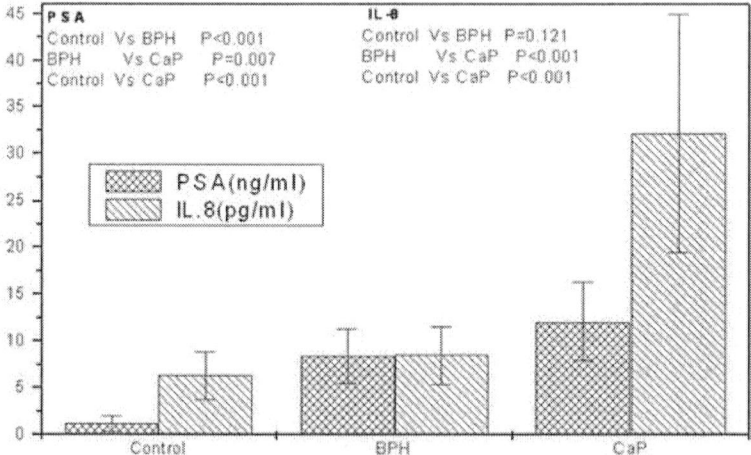

Figure 1. Serum Levels of pro-angiogenic chemokine IL-8 in prostate cancer patients compared to normal and benign prostatic hyperplasia Patients.

TGF-β has been shown to be pro-angiogenic *in vivo*, and over-expression of TGF-β in tumor cells can result in tumor growth and metastasis [106,107]. The effect of TGF-β is biphasic; at lower concentrations, it promotes VEGF expression and basic fibroblast growth factor induced epithelial tubule formation, while at higher concentrations, it inhibits these activities. TGF-β over production also has been shown to favor malignancy by suppression of the cellular and humoral immunity of the host, promotion of angiogenesis, stimulation of stromal matrix formation, and enhancement of prostate cancer cell motility and metastasis [108]. Of the various isoforms of TGF-β, TGF-β1, which was purified initially from the PC-3 metastatic human CaP cell line [109], was believed to inhibit proliferation of normal prostatic epithelial cells. However, with malignant transformation, prostate cancer cells over-express TGF-β1 and become resistant to its growth inhibitory effects [110]. Although numerous studies on the relationship between TGF-β1 and prostate cancer have been reported, there are only limited and conflicting reports on the association with prostate cancer of the other isoform, TGF-β2. Several studies have shown that TGF-β2 mRNA and protein are overproduced by the PC-3 and LNCaP prostate cancer cell lines [109,111], while other studies have reported that TGF-β2 mRNA levels are unchanged in prostate cancer compared to benign tissue [111,112]. However, in a clinical study where patients with prostate cancer were grouped by pathological stage or Gleason grade, plasma TGF-β2 levels were highest in patients with low pathological stages and low-grade disease, suggesting that TGF-β2 may be associated with the degree of tumor differentiation.

In an attempt to identify underlying differences in the secretory pattern of cytokines and growth factors involved in angiogenesis, and to correlate the differences in constitutive expression of these genes with the metastatic potential of prostate cancer cell lines, we under took a study using three different prostate cancer cell lines LNCaP, DU-145 and PC-3 characterized as possessing low, moderate, and high metastatic potential, as demonstrated by their differential capacity to invade an extracellular matrix, an established tumor invasion assay [73]. Cells were cultured for 48 h, RNA was extracted and amplified by PCR, and the amplified products were run on 1.2% agarose gel. Figure 2*A* presents the constitutive level of gene expression of select pro-angiogeneic growth factors. VEGF mRNA levels were significantly higher in PC-3 and DU-145 cells as compared with the weakly metastatic LNCaP cells. VEGF expression by DU-145 and PC-3 cells, respectively, was 3- and 5-fold greater than LNCaP cells (Figure 2B, *a*). mRNA levels of other pro-angiogenic factors, such as TGF-β2, IL-8, and ICAM-1, also were considerably greater in the highly metastatic cell line, PC-3, and in the moderately metastatic DU-145 cells, compared with LNCaP cells (Figure 2*A*, *rows 3–5*, and Figure 2B, *b–d*). In contrast, constitutive expression of IFN-γ mRNA, (Figure 2*A*, *row 6*) was highest in the poorly metastatic LNCaP cells (Figure 2B, *e*). IFN-γ in LNCaP was significantly greater ($P < 0.001$) than the constitutive gene expression in DU-145 (Figure 2*A*, *row 6, Lane 3*) and PC-3 (Figure 2*A*, *row 6, Lane 4*) cells. To determine whether the patterns of gene expression of angiogenic factors were reflected at the protein level, equal aliquots of culture supernatants, harvested from the same number (3×10^6) of cells, were assayed using a sandwich ELISA procedure. DU-145 and PC-3 cells secreted VEGF at levels that were 2- and 4-fold higher, respectively, than LNCaP cells (Figure 2C, *a*). TGF-β2 levels in supernatants from PC-3 (404 ± 27 pg/ml) and DU-145 (385 ± 25 pg/ml) cells also were significantly higher ($P < 0.001$ for both) than levels in LNCaP supernatants (4.0 ± 0.8; Figure 2C, *b*). Because angiogenesis and metastasis also are associated with IL-8 and ICAM-1 expression, we measured the amounts of these products secreted into culture supernatants. The concentration of IL-8 in the conditioned medium of PC-3 cells after 48 h of culture was 185 ± 18 pg/ml, which was significantly higher ($P < 0.001$) than for LNCaP cells (25 ± 20 pg/ml), but not significantly different from the amount secreted by DU-145 cells (175 ± 18 pg/ml). Furthermore, secreted levels of ICAM-1 protein also were significantly higher in the supernatants of DU-145 and PC-3 cells, (24.0 ± 5.0 and 38.0 ± 7.0 pg/ml, respectively) ($P < 0.001$ for both), when compared with the conditioned medium of LNCaP cells (4.0 ± 0.8 pg/ml). In contrast, LNCaP cells secreted significantly more IFN-γ protein (~2-fold more) than the highly Metastatic PC-3 cells (Figure 2C, *e*), consistent with the differential expression of IFN-γ mRNA. The observed differences in gene or protein expression were not correlated with variation in viability or rate of cell growth.

The gene expression results of the Northern analyses were confirmed using quantitative, real-time reverse transcription-PCR, and included normal prostate epithelial cells as standards for comparison with the prostate cancer cell lines (Figure 2D). When compared with normal prostate epithelial cells, the prostate cancer cell lines demonstrated consistently higher levels of expression of the genes for a wide range of pro-angiogenic factors. Moreover expression of these genes positively correlated with the metastatic potential of the cell line (i.e., expression of pro-angiogenic genes by PC-3 > DU-145 > LNCaP). As expected for normal cells, benign prostate epithelial cells did not show significant expression of the IFN-γ gene. In conclusion, our study [73] for the first time documented that constitutive expression of the mRNA for pro-angiogenic factors, VEGF, ICAM-1, IL-8, and TGF-β2, was significantly greater in the more metastatic DU-145 and PC-3 prostate cancer cells compared with LNCaP cells. In addition, protein levels of VEGF, ICAM-1, and IL-8 were significantly higher in the metastatic PC-3 and DU-145 prostate cancer cell lines compared with LNCaP cells. Conversely, gene expression and protein synthesis of the anti-angiogenic factor IFN-γ was significantly decreased in the moderately metastatic DU-145 cells, and highly metastatic PC-3 cells, compared with the poorly metastatic LNCaP cells, providing evidence for the first time for a link between the metastatic potential of CaP cells and their expression of several factors that modulate angiogenesis [73].

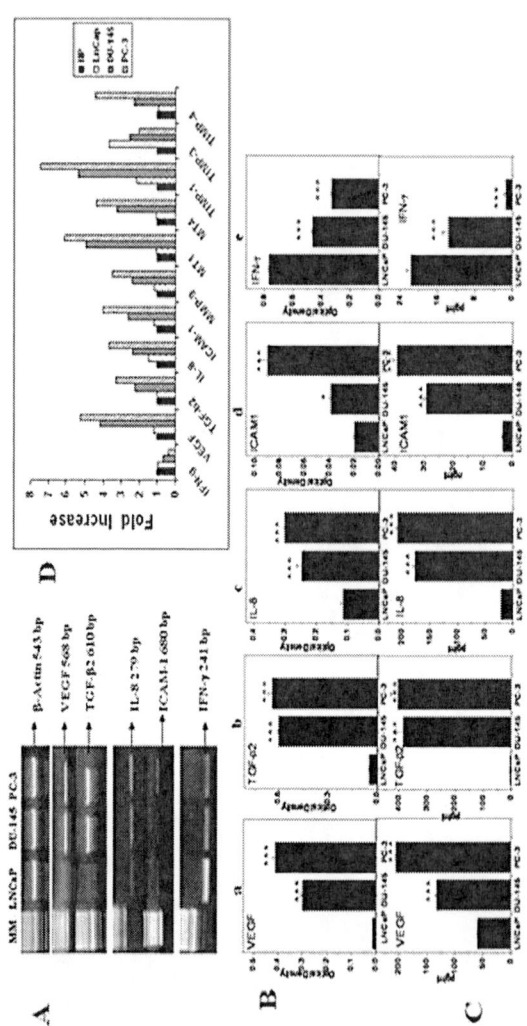

Figure 2. Constitutive expression of pro- and anti-angiogenic factors by normal prostate epithelial cells (NP) and prostate cancer cell lines of low (LNCaP), moderate (DU-145), high (PC-3) invasive potential. A) Agarose gel electrophoresis profiles of the PCR amplimers of pro- and anti-angiogenic factors. B) Mean densitometric values of bands in A. C) Levels of angiogenic factors secreted into the culture supernatant. D) Quantitative real-time (Q)PCR analysis of pro- and anti-angiogenic genes expressed as fold increase in ΔCT compared to normal prostate epithelial cells as unity. Normal prostate epithelial or tumor cells (3×10^6) were cultured for 48 hr, RNA was extracted and subjected to QPCR using specific primers, including the housekeeping gene, β-actin. Amplified PCR products were electrophoresed on an agarose gel containing ethidium bromide and confirmed by QPCR. Culture supernates were assayed for angiogenic factors by ELISA. Values are the mean ± SE of 4 experiments. *, $P<0.05$ and ***, $P<0.001$ when compared to LNCaP cells.

Chapter VI

Role of PSA in CaP Angiogenesis

Despite the importance of PSA as a surrogate marker for early detection of prostate cancer, or of treatment failure, relatively few studies have addressed the physiological function of PSA and its relation to the pathogenesis and progression of prostate cancer. The most widely accepted physiological function of PSA is the liquefication of the seminal coagulum. More recently, attention has been drawn to PSA as a regulatory molecule in prostate tumor growth and metastasis. There are several reports that demonstrate PSA has anti-tumorigenic and anti-angiogenic activity. We have shown that prostate cancer cell lines that vary in their metastatic potential demonstrate differential expression of growth factors that control tumor growth and metastasis, and of PSA [73]. The highly metastatic human prostate cancer cell line PC-3M has higher expression of growth factors like VEGF, IL-8, TGF-β2, ICAM-1 and MMP-9 that are known to promote tumor growth compared to LNCaP cells that are poorly metastatic, and that produce low levels of PSA [73]. Incubation of prostate cancer cells with PSA caused the release of anti-angiogenic fragments (angiostatin-like) by proteolytic digestion of extra-cellular matrix components and plasminogen [114]. Both enzymatically active and inactive forms of PSA had anti-angiogenic activity *in vitro* in the Matrigel tube formation assay [115]. Consistent with an anti-angiogenic potential, we reported that purified enzymatically active, as well as inactive, free PSA (f-PSA is not complexed with carrier proteins) down-regulated expression of pro-angiogenic growth factors/cancer genes/proteins, including VEGF, IL-8, EphA2, CYR61, Bcl2, Pim-1 oncogene, and uPA, and up-regulated expression of anti-angiogenic genes/proteins, including IFN and IFN-related genes in treated cancer cells [116]. In addition, we demonstrated that f-PSA inhibited growth of the PC-3M prostate tumor xenograft in nude mice [116]. Our data suggested strongly that enzymatic activity of PSA was not essential for its effect on gene expression, anti-angiogenic activity and anti-tumor activity [116]. However, Mattsson et al [117] reported recently that recombinant pro-PSA does not demonstrate anti-angiogenic activity. However, the unprocessed pro-protein used in these studies that due to structural differences from the proteolytically activated mature PSA protein, may not be an appropriate control for mature PSA protein in which enzymatic activity is blocked.

Chapter VII

Isolation and Characterization of Human PSA for Evaluation of the Physiological Role of PSA in Angiogenesis

The role PSA during the onset of prostate cancer development, and subsequent tumor progression and metastasis, is not well understood. As reviewed in the previous section, PSA has been documented as an anti-angiogenic molecule and an inducer of apoptosis [115,118]. PSA has been shown to inhibit endothelial cell proliferation, migration and invasion [118], and inhibits endothelial cell responses to FGF-2 and VEGF that are known to stimulate angiogenesis [118]. These observations collectively support the idea that PSA may have a role in prostate tumor growth and metastasis. In order to critically assess the role of PSA as a "biomarker", or as a "therapeutic modality", it is critical to have a high quality source of PSA that is well characterized and enzymatically active. Although expression of cloned PSA has been reported [119], it is critical that PSA from a natural source should be used initially for assessing its physiological functions. We were the first group to establish a simple two-step procedure that allows isolation of enzymatically active f-PSA from seminal plasma with high over all recovery [39]. The availability of isolated high purity enzymatically active f-PSA will facilitate evaluation of the physiological role(s) of PSA in prostate tumor cell proliferation, migration and metastasis. Briefly, the two step procedure for isolation of PSA is based on principles of hydrophobic charge-induction chromatography and molecular size chromatography, and yields pure free-

PSA (f-PSA) preparations free from all other known PSA complexes and human kallikrein 2 (hK2). The overall recovery of f-PSA by this method was 72%. The isolated f-PSA consisted of three known isoforms that correspond to *pIs* of 6.2, 6.4 and 7.2 f-PSA, are enzymatically active, and demonstrate enzymatic activity that is effectively neutralized by serine protease inhibitors [39].

Table 1. Amino-terminal sequence of f-PSA from (seminal plasma)

^{25}Ile-Val-Gly-Gly-Trp-Cys-Glu-Lys-His-Full Length

^{26}Val-Gly-Gly-Trp-Glu-Cys-X-Lys-His-Ser-N-1

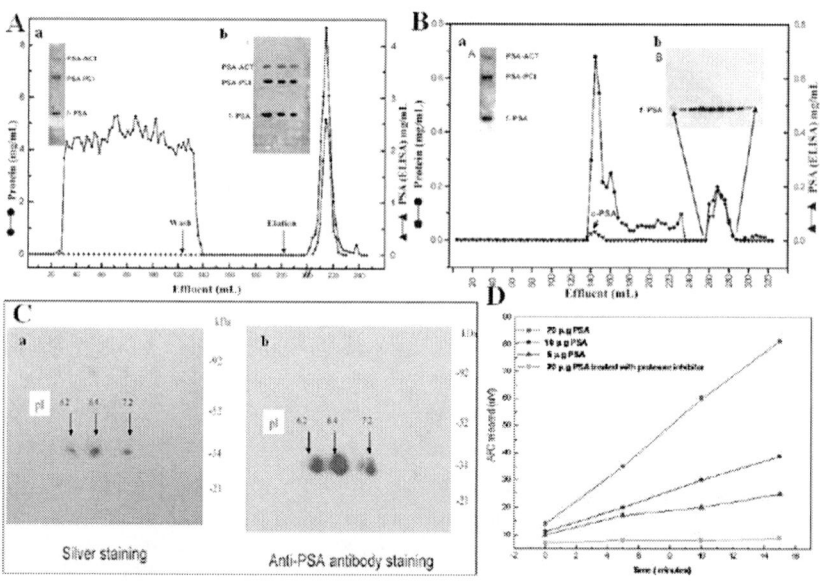

Figure 3. Isolation and characterization of human PSA from Seminal Plasma. (A)Chromatography of seminal plasma on Fractogel TA650s. The column was equilibrated with 25mM Hepes buffer containing 1M sodium sulfate, pH 7.0. Seminal plasma was dialyzed against column equilibrating buffer and applied to the column. The column was washed and the bound proteins were eluted with 25mM Hepes buffer. The protein concentration was measured by BCA method and PSA was monitored by either SDS/PAGE Western-blot analysis using monoclonal anti-PSA antibody or by

double determined ELISA. Insert: (a) PSA isoforms (f-PSA, PSA–PCI and PSA–ACT) present in the starting material. The presence of PSA–PCI and PSA–ACT was subsequently confirmed by monoclonal antibodies to PCI and ACT. (b) All three PSA isoforms were recovered in the column eluates. (B) Chromatography of T-gel processed seminal proteins on Ultrogel AcA-54 column. The column was equilibrated with 10mM sodium acetate buffer containing 0.15Msodium chloride, pH 5.6. The concentrated seminal proteins, after T-gel chromatography and containing f-PSA, PSA–PCI and PSA–ACT and other proteins were applied to the column. The column was developed at the flow rate of 16 ml/h and 4ml fractions were collected. The protein was monitored by the BCA protein assay procedure. PSA presence was monitored either by SDS/PAGE Western-blot analysis using anti-PSA antibody or quantitated by the double determined ELISA using anti-PSA antibodies. Insert: (a) f-PSA, PSA–PCI and PSA–ACT in the starting material. (b) f-PSA. (C) 2-D gel electrophoresis of f-PSA. The blots were developed either with silver stain (a) or by chemiluminescent agent after probing the membrane with anti-PSA antibody (b). Three distinct spots were seen corresponding to pI 6.2, 6.4 and 7.2. The identical spots were llluminated in both gels. Beside PSA isoforms, no other proteins were detected in gel stained with silver nitrate. (D) Enzymatic activity of f-PSA. The reaction mixture contained 10 μl of 20mM concentration of highly specific chromogenic substrate and varying concentrations of f-PSA (5, 10 and 20 μg) in total of 500 μl of 50mM Tris.HCl, pH 7.9 buffer. The amount of AFC released over a period of time was monitored using Aminco-Bowman Spectrophotometer. There is a dose dependent increase in amount of AFC released by increasing concentration of f-PSA. The enzymatic activity of f-PSA was completely blocked when f-PSA was exposed to a serine protease inhibitor, Aprotinin before being exposed to the substrate.

Chapter VIII

Purification and Characterization of f-PSA from Seminal Plasma

A simple two step chromatographic procedure was validated for purification and isolation of enzymatically active f-PSA from human seminal plasma [39,120,121]. The initial step involves separation of PSA from the bulk of non-PSA proteins in seminal plasma by Thiophilic Charge Induction chromatography [Fractogel TA 650s (T-gel); EM Sciences, Gibbstown, NJ, USA]. T-gel has a strong affinity for all molecular forms of PSA, including both free and complexed. Seminal plasma was dialyzed against column equilibration buffer (25 mM HEPES, pH 7.0, containing 1.0 M Na_2SO_4) and was applied to the T-gel column. Approximately 10% of seminal plasma proteins are retained on the T-gel column. Bound proteins (free and complexed PSA and immunoglobulins) were displaced from the column by lowering the salt concentration of the elution buffer (Figure 3A). PSA recovery was >90%. The presence of PSA and PSA-complexes in the eluate was confirmed by western-blot analysis using antibodies specific to PSA, and to the three serine proteinase inhibitors in serum that are known to form complexes with PSA: alpha-1 antichymotrypsin (ACT), alpha-2 macroglobulin (α_2M) and Protein-C inhibitor (PCI) (Figure 3B, a). Subsequently, f-PSA was separated completely from complexed-PSA using Molecular Size Chromatography on Ultrogel AcA54 (Biosepra, Freemont, CA). PSA eluted from the T-gel column was concentrated (Amicon PM-10 membrane) and applied to an Ultrogel AcA54 column (2.5x100 cm) equilibrated with 10 mM sodium phosphate buffer, pH 7.0. The fractions containing f-PSA were identified using western-blot analysis with an anti-PSA antibody (Figure 3B, b), and the fractions containing f-PSA were pooled, concentrated using PM10 membranes (Amicon) and filter sterilized. Quantitation of f-PSA was performed by a sandwich ELISA, using commercially available PSA as a standard, the concentration of PSA adjusted to 1-3 mg/ml, and the aliquots frozen at −70°C. Purity of the isolated f-PSA was verified by silver-staining/antibody staining of 2-D gels (Figure 3C, a, b), and the purified f-PSA was characterized for enzymatic activity using a fluorogenic substrate specific for PSA (Figure 3D) [122]. The average yield of f-PSA is 0.5 mg/ml of seminal plasma. Our procedure is milder and avoids any denaturing conditions. The use of thiophilic-gel chromatography as a first step in purification procedure allows processing of large volume of seminal plasma as this column matrix retains <10% of the seminal plasma protein applied. The matrix has high capacity (10–15 mg protein/ml adsorbent) and can be used both in a standard column chromatography format and in a batch adsorption format. PSA complexes and other high molecular weight proteins, including immunoglobulins, were separated from f-PSA during the second column step based on gel filtration chromatography, on an AcA54 column. The AcA54 column was developed in a buffer at pH 7.0 to avoid auto cleavage of PSA during purification. The overall recovery of purified f-PSA ranged between 64 and 78% of total PSA present in the starting material. This represents a significant improvement in overall PSA recovery from reported previously. The average recoveries reported in the literature ranged between 7 and 30% of total PSA [123-125]. In majority of these reports, PSA recovery was characterized either by SDS/PAGE or by amino-terminal sequencing, and not by enzymatic activity. The immunological characterization of PSA was based upon mono- and polyclonal antibodies to PSA in SDS/PAGE/Western-blot analyses. The purity of f-PSA preparations were confirmed initially by 2-D gel electrophoresis, with protein bands visualized by silver staining or by immunostaining with monoclonal anti-PSA antibodies. Importantly, PSA has been demonstrated to exist in multiple isoforms [124,126], with the variability due to differences in either the primary structure of the protein or in the pattern of glycosylation. We have identified three isoforms of f-PSA with p*Is of* 6.2, 6.4 and 7.2. These three isoforms were consistently seen in different preparations of f-PSA purified from seminal plasma. Definitive sequence identification of two PSA isoforms was established based on N-terminal sequence data (Table 1): one sequence corresponded to full length PSA and the other corresponded to a PSA protein that lacked the isoleucine residue at position N1. The full length sequence was enzymatically active, whereas, the N−1 sequence had no enzymatic activity [115]. The third PSA isoform (<10 kDa) represented <5%

of total f-PSA and was observed occasionally. This sequence was not present initially in our f-PSA preparations because the second step in our purification involved a molecular sizing step that effectively separated the low molecular weight PSA sequences from the full length sequence. Alternatively, this protein might be generated as an artifact due to storage and/or handling of f-PSA. The PSA gene (hK3) is a member of the human tissue kallikrein gene family that consists of at least three well characterized members [127]. Seminal plasma is known to have both human kallikrein-2 (hK2) and human kallikrein-3 (hK3) proteins. Because of extensive sequence homology between these two kallikrein, it is conceivable that our f-PSA preparation from the Thiophilic gel separation may have traces of hK2. However, the probability of hK2 contamination in the f-PSA preparation is very low since in seminal plasma, hK2 level is 80–500-fold lower than hK3. The reported value of hk3 in seminal plasma ranges from 0.5–3.0 mg/ml [123,128], whereas and that of hK2 is 6.0 µg/ml [129]. Furthermore, essentially all hK2 present in the seminal plasma is complexed with PCI [130] and the complex is of much higher molecular weight than f-PSA. which can be effectively eliminated in the second purification step. f-PSA purified by our protocol is enzymatically active (Figure 3D): the enzymatic activity is dose dependent, and was blocked by serine protease inhibitors (SERPIN) (Figure 3D). PSA enzymatic activity was associated with complete amino acid sequence, that lack of the N-terminal isoleucine destroys its enzymatic activity [131]. In our preparations, 70% of f-PSA was enzymatically active (in agreement with earlier reports [132]).

Chapter IX

Role of f-PSA in Angiogenesis and Prostate Tumor Growth: Gene Expression Profile

Microarray technology as a "gene discovery tool" has identified genetic markers that discriminate between normal and cancerous tissues. Gene expression profiles of expression of thousands of genes in normal and prostate tumor tissues have been used in hierarchical clustering analysis to sort specimens [133,134]. Dhanasekaran, et.al., [134] were able to distinguish normal prostate, BPH, localized prostate cancer and metastatic prostate cancer samples using microarrays. Using hierarchical clustering analysis, Luo *et al.* [135] were able to discriminate 16 prostate cancer samples from nine BPH specimens on the basis of differences in gene expression profiles. Hence, we used gene array technology and Real Time PCR to study the regulatory effect of enzymatically active f-PSA on gene expression in prostate cancer cell lines. f-PSA purified to homogeneity from human seminal plasma by column chromatography, eliminating hk2 and all known PSA complexes yet retaining its protease activity, was applied to confluent monolayers of the CaP cell lines PC-3M and LNCaP, to determine changes in expression of various genes known to regulate angiogenesis, tumor growth and metastasis. PSA induced significant changes in expression of various cancer-related genes in PC-3M and LNCaP cells. In a gene array analysis of PC-3M cells treated with 10 mM f-PSA, 136 genes were up regulated and 137 genes were down regulated [136]. In LNCaP cells treated with an identical concentration of f-PSA, a total of 793 genes were differentially regulated [136]. QPCR analysis revealed that the genes for urokinase-type plasminogen activator (uPA), VEGF, and Pim-1 oncogene were significantly down-regulated, whereas, IFN-γ, known to be a tumor-suppressor gene, was significantly up regulated in f-PSA–treated PC-3M cells [136]. The effect of f-PSA on VEGF and IFN-γ gene expression, and on protein release in PC-3M cells, was distinctly dose-dependent [136]. To verify the results with an *in vivo* model, PC-3M cells subcutaneously injected into athymic nude mice were selected and the animals were treated with f-PSA. The tumors were treated with 150 μg f-PSA three times a week, and tumor growth was followed for four weeks. Tumor in control animals were evident at the inoculated site by two weeks, while tumors in PSA treated mice were not palpable. Tumor volume and tumor weight of the f-PSA treated mice were significantly lower than that of the control animals at all time points (Figure 4 A& B). Tumor volume in PSA treated animals by the end of 4 weeks was 267.2 mm^3, whereas, that of the control animal was 423.9 mm^3 ($p = 0.038$) (Figure 4A). The mean tumor weight of the treated mice was 420 mg while that of the control animals was 767 mg ($p= 0.03$) (Figure 4B). Treatment of PC-3M tumor with f-PSA produced a significant reduction in the tumor progression. Tumor volume measured by f-MRI imaging was significantly different in PSA treated versus control treated animals (Figure 4C) suggesting purified PSA had marked anti-tumor properties.

Mechanistically, the anti-tumor action of PSA was presumed to be due to its serine protease activity. However, complexing of PSA with ACT not only blocked the enzymatic activity, but also blocked its anti-angiogenic property [118]. However it has also been reported that both the full length PSA (enzymatically active) and the N-1 variant (enzymatically inactive) have anti-angiogenic property. It strongly implies that PSA can exert its anti-tumor activity by multiple mechanisms. Our study documented, for the first time, that enzymatically active/inactive f-PSA (inhibited by zinc) was 99.9% pure and significantly modulates gene/protein expression of several pro and anti angiogenic growth factors [136]. This suggests that enzymatic activity of PSA is not required for its anti angiogenic property.

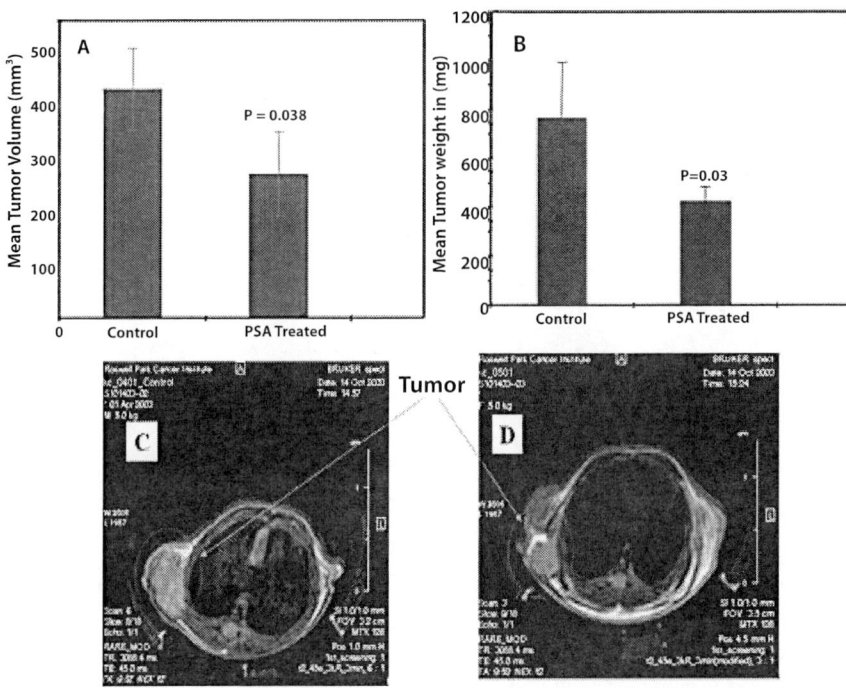

Figure 4. Effect of f-PSA treatment of PC-3M tumor-bearing nude mice on tumor volume and weight. Five-week – old male athymic BALB/c nude mice were injected subcutaneously with 1×10^6 PC-3M tumor cells in the neck region, assigned to either control (treated with PBS injections administered subcutaneously within the tumor vicinity and on alternate days for a total of 4 weeks) or f-PSA – treated groups (150µg of f-PSA administered subcutaneously within the tumor vicinity and on alternate days for a total of 4 weeks), sacrificed at the end of 4 weeks. Both tumor volume and tumor weights were measured for each animal. There were five animals in each group. Average tumor volume (A), average tumor weight (B), tumor growth monitored by f-MRI in control at 4 weeks [mean tumor volume = 424 mm^3] (C) and tumor growth monitored by f-MRI in f-PSA treated at 4 weeks [mean tumor volume = 267 mm^3] (D). Both tumor volume and tumor weight were significantly reduced in PSA treated animals.

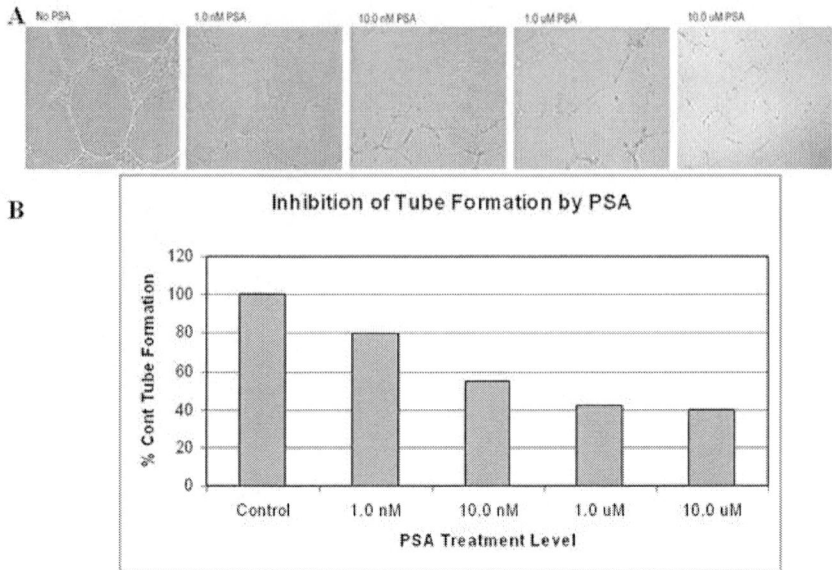

Figure 5. Inhibition of "Angiogenesis" in the HUVEC Matrigel Tube Formation Assay. HUVEC cells were cultured in a medium optimized for endothelial cells that is supplemented with low serum (2%) to preferentially favor proliferation of endothelial cells and select against proliferation of stromal and myoepithelial cells either without, or with f-PSA at different doses. Biological effects of putative anti-angiogenic agents were evaluated by the reduction in area occupied by "tube" structures in the culture, or by measurement of the length of the tube structures determined by placing axes within the structures and summing the lengths of the axes. (A) Representative image of Tube formation by HUVEC cells on Matrigel (B) Quantative analysis of inhibition of Tube formation by PSA. Automated quantitation of area, or axis lengths, was performed by digital image analysis using OPTIMAS or ImagePro.

Chapter X

Role of PSA in Angiogenesis by Endothelial Cells *In Vitro*

As mentioned earlier, PSA has been reported to have anti-angiogenic activity [115,118]. Transfection of PSA c-DNA into PC-3 prostate cancer cells prolonged doubling time, induced apoptosis, and reduced tumorogenicity and metastasis in nude mice [113]. In addition, PSA released anti-angiogenic fragments (angiostatin-like) by proteolytic digestion of extra-cellular matrix components and plasminogen [114]. However, both enzymatically active and inactive forms of PSA have been shown to have anti-angiogenic activity *in vitro* and *in vivo* [115]. Consistent with these reports, we have shown that both purified enzymatically active and inactive, f-PSA down-regulated expression of pro-angiogenic and growth related genes in PC-3 cells, including VEGF, EphA2, CYR61, Bcl2, Pim-1 oncogene, and uPA, and up-regulated expression of anti-angiogenic genes/proteins, including interferon and interferon-related genes [116] and peptide inhibitors of angiogeneis. Formation of tube-like structures in Matrigel by HUVEC is a well characterized *in vitro* assay of "angiogenic" activity that has been utilized extensively to evaluate *in vitro* the anti-angiogenic capacity of peptides, proteins and pharmacologic agents [137,138]. We analyzed the effects of f-PSA on HUVEC to better understand the role of f-PSA in the modulation of angiogenesis. In our study purified f-PSA was mixed with liquid Matrigel, ten thousand HUVEC cells were added to the liquefied Matrigel, the cell suspension plated in a well of a 24-well tissue culture plate, and the assay incubated for 24 hours for tube formation. In the absence of PSA, HUVECs efficiently migrated, coalesced and formed tube-like structures during the 24 hr incubation. In contrast, PSA inhibited significantly, in a dose dependent manner, the migration/chemotaxsis and attachment functions required for tube formation by HUVEC. Figure 5A provides a quantitative summary, and Figure 5B is a graphic representation of the dose-related inhibition of HUVEC's tubular structure formation by f-PSA in Matrigel.

Chapter XI

Effect of Treatment of CaP Cells (PC-3M) with f-PSA on the Differential Expression of Proteins

While the physiological activity of PSA in liquefying the seminal clot is well understood, its role in the micro/macro-environment of the prostate, including its effects on prostate cancer progression, remains to be elucidated. Considerable research analyzing gene expression at the transcriptional level is ongoing in cancer cells. However, this approach is limited as mRNA levels do not necessarily correlate with translation to the respective protein. Furthermore, post-translational modification of proteins by proteolysis, recycling and protein-protein interactions cannot be detected by gene expression assays. Since f-PSA is obtained in sufficient quantities using the methodology described above, and the powerful new technology of proteomics can differentiate proteins expressed under normal and disease states, we used a combination of these approaches to study the effect of PSA on protein expression in prostate cancer cells. The effect of PSA on protein expression at the level of the entire proteome were analyzed using 2D-DIGE coupled with LC–MS/MS. Using purified f-PSA we analyzed *in vitro* the effect of f-PSA on the proteomes of the prostate cancer cell, PC-3M. PC-3M cells were treated with 10 mM f-PSA for 48 hr. The time course and concentration of f-PSA chosen were based on our prior experience, and concentrations reported by others in the literature. Protein samples from six different PC-3M cell lysates were labeled with fluorescent dyes, pooled, and analyzed in triplicate by 2D-

DIGE. The DIA (differential in-gel analysis) module of the differential analysis software DeCyder (GE healthcare) was used to calculate protein spot volumes, and normalized volume ratio, for each differentially labeled protein spot that co-migrated.. The ratio of spot intensity with, and without, PSA treatment followed a near normal distribution with about 12% of the proteins down-regulated and 4% of the proteins up-regulated by PSA. Gel to gel matching of the standard spot maps from each gel was performed using the DeCyder BVA software module. This allowed for the statistical analysis of changes in protein abundance between samples. Statistical analysis (paired t-test) was performed for the difference between the abundance of proteins from untreated PC-3M cells versus proteins from f-PSA treated PC-3M cells. A total of 41 protein spots out of an average 2,250 spots showed a significant change in abundance ($P<0.05$), and thirty of these spots were then selected in the order of the significance of their respective volume ratios for further analysis by nano-high performance liquid chromatography followed by tandem mass spectrometry (nano-LC–MS/MS). Proteins from 26 gel spots were successfully identified. Figure 6, is the SYPRO Ruby stained 2D gel image showing all protein spots. Differentially expressed protein spots showing significant modulation in response to incubation with PSA were selected for subsequent identification and are shown as numbered outlines. The maximum increase in protein expression was 1.66-fold (spot 508 in Figure 6A), and the maximum decrease observed was 2.2-fold (spot #600, Figure 6A). The highest molecular weight of the proteins analyzed was 61 kDa. Figure 6B, shows the change in expression of a unique protein spot (#600) from the 2D-DIGE analysis of untreated PC-3M cells (Figure 6B) in comparison with cells treated for 48 hr with 10 mM f-PSA (Figure 6C). Of all the protein spots examined, spot #600 manifested the greatest change in expression, showing a 2.16-fold down-regulation ($P=0.0001$). Quantitation of the abundance of spot #600 in untreated and treated PC-3M cells is depicted in Figure 6D and E, respectively. Figure 6F shows that the gel to gel variation of spot intensities between untreated (Group I) and treated (Group II) PC-3M cells from three separate experiments were negligible. Spots were picked robotically from the SYPRO Ruby stained gels as designated by a vertical bar (Figure 6D and E) and were digested with trypsin. The resultant peptides were separated by nano-HPLC and the eluted peptides were directed into a Thermo-Finnigan LCQDecaXPPlus ion-trap mass spectrometer providing the mass analysis of the fragments. The mass range scanned was 0–1500 amu. Figure 6F shows the unique MS/MS analysis spectra of the tryptic peptide, ASAFSSVGSVITK, obtained from spot #600 which was subsequently identified as the N8 gene long isoform. Other significantly down-regulated proteins were: heat shock protein beta-1 (Hspb1, 2.13-fold, P=0.021), peroxiredoxin- 6 (2.13-fold, P=0.021), tri-phospolipase isomerase-1 (1.92-fold, P=0.043), laminin receptor 1 (1.74-fold, P=0.0052), nucleolar phosphoprotein B23.2 (1.64-fold, P=0.0085), heat shock protein 60 (Hsp60, 1.58-fold, P=0.028), apoptosis inhibitor FKSG2 (1.52-fold, P=0.023), and oncogene DJ1 (1.49-fold,P=0.027). Proteins that were up-regulated by f-PSA treatment included: tumor protein D54 (1.66-fold, P=0.047), ubiquinol–cytochrome c reductase binding protein (1.54-fold, P=0.045), human platelet profilin (1.44-fold, P=0.023), heterogenous nuclear ribonucleoprotein G (1.66-fold, P=0.023), and human platelet profilin complexed with the L-pro10 peptide (1.2-fold, P=0.027). Table 2 (down-regulated proteins) and Table 3 (upregulated proteins) list all identified proteins, their gene accession number, percentage of the sequence identified, and their physiological significance. Among these proteins, laminin receptor, GAPDH, and DJ1 specifically have been linked to prostate cancer [144,145]. The N8 gene product long isoform was observed to undergo the greatest extent of down-regulation (2.2-fold) upon treatment of PC-3M cells with f-PSA. The N8 gene is highly expressed in tumors, including prostate cancer [146]. Laminins are a family of extracellular matrix proteins that constitute the major non-collagenous glycoproteins found in the basement membrane and are involved in multiple biological activities [147] including, cell attachment [147,148], migration [147,149], growth and differentiation [148] and angiogenesis [148,150]. The interaction of cancer cells with laminin is a key event in tumor invasion and metastasis [147,151,152]. One of the mechanisms by which laminin contributes to the metastatic spread of cancer is induction of proteolytic activity. In certain malignant, but not in normal cells, laminin induces an increase in matrix metalloproteinase-2 (MMP-2) activity [153]. MMP-2 is an extracellular, matrix-degrading endopeptidase, which plays a key role in invasion and metastasis and is frequently correlated with tumor progression [154]. Up-regulation of the laminin receptor correlates with enhanced invasiveness and metastatic potential in many malignancies [155,156]. The laminin receptor has been implicated in laminin-induced tumor cell attachment [156] and migration [149], as well as in tumor angiogenesis [148], growth, invasion and metastasis [157]. In our analysis of the proteome of f-PSA treated PC-3M cells we documented that laminin receptor 1 is down-regulated (Table 2). The relevance of the level of PSA in the prostate cancer tissue microenvironment, and its relation to tumor progression, have not been elucidated. Our observation that at physiologic concentrations f-PSA down-regulates expression of multiple proteins known to have involvement in tumor progression suggests that a role for PSA in prostate tissue microenvironment is the maintenance of a non-angiogenic environment, and that down-regulation of PSA expression with progression or androgen deprivation therapy may promote tumor growth.

As a follow up to our analyses of the proteome changes induced by PSA, we performed a biological network analysis using the Metacore pathway mapping tool to map the common, biological pathways that contained the differentially expressed proteins. The algorithm builds biological networks from the list of differentially expressed proteins, and assigns a biological process to each network. Proteins differentially expressed in response to treatment with f-PSA were primarily involved in the following processes: intracellular signaling, cell differentiation, response to stress, neoplastic events, regulation of apoptosis, and cell death. The significance of associations between the biological processes and the differentially expressed proteins are represented by P-values. The cellular processes that showed highly significant association with the differentially expressed proteins included: apoptosis (P-value=9.16×10^{-17}), cell death (P=3.42×10^{-15}), regulation of apoptosis (P =3.33×10^{-8}), and response to stress (P= 2.3×10^{-12}). Significant association of these proteins with pathologic processes (P=2.8×10^{-10}), neoplastic processes (P=1.8×10^{-8}) and neuro-ectodermal tumors (P=1.12×10^{-8}) suggest that they may be biomarkers for prostate cancer. Figure 7 illustrates the close clustering and inter-connectedness of the biochemical process networks modulated by PSA. The clustering network was generated using the shortest path algorithm to map interaction between the proteins. Nodes represent the individual proteins, and lines between nodes indicate direct protein-protein interactions. Highlighted lines represent specific, designated pathways, and background lines represent secondary, related biological pathways. Proteins identified in the MS/MS analyses as modulated by PSA are denoted by a circle around the nodes. Figure 7A represents a highlighted network relating neoplastic events, and Figure 7B represents processes involving regulation of apoptosis and cell death. A network generated by merging cellular processes involved in intracellular signaling cascades, cell differentiation, and cell stress responses integrates most of the proteins identified in these pathways (Figure 7C).

Data analyses using MetaCore's manually curated database show that many of the proteins down-regulated in PC-3M cells by treatment with f-PSA, are involved directly or indirectly, in the p53 pathway. Figure 7 shows various networks generated from MetaCore's extensive annotated content database using various network creating algorithms. Some of the genes are connected by association with other objects, including transcription factors (e.g., p53), binding proteins (e.g., caspase), receptors, enzymes (e.g., kinases, phosphatases, proteases, and GTPases), and co-regulated genes. Therefore, nodes that contain connections to large numbers of root objects represent key regulators, and the shortest path algorithm maps the interactions among these differentially expressed proteins. One of the most prominent regulatory proteins common to these networks is p53, in that it interacts with several of the differentially expressed proteins, including Hsp60, LAMR1, and vimentin that are involved in neoplastic events. A merged network diagram of processes, including intercellular signaling cascades, cell differentiation and stress responses is depicted in Figure 7C. This demonstrates that most of the identified proteins whose expression was significantly modulated by PSA are directly, or indirectly, involved in these processes. In addition, other transcription factors (p53, androgen receptor, ESR2, and STAT5), also were identified in these networks, suggesting their potential role in prostate cancer biology. The data illustrated in Figure 7 also suggest that the interaction of Hsp60 and p53 is mediated via Bcl-xL. It is known that over-expression of Hsp60 increases the abundance of the anti-apoptotic Bcl-xL gene product, and reduces the protein expression of the pro-apoptotic BAX gene [158]. Bcl-xL, in turn, inhibits p53-dependent apoptosis by sequestering cytoplasmic p53, preventing it from activating BAX [159]. Identification of p53 as a key player in many of the networks suggests that it may participate in the transcriptional activation of multiple key pathways common in prostate cancer. The proteins Hsp27 and NPM/ALK that are down-regulated by PSA, as shown in Figure 7B and C, are known to contribute to cancer progression. The phosphorylated dimer of Hsp27 interacts with Daxx, preventing its subsequent interaction with Ask1 and Fas, thus blocking Daxx-mediated apoptosis. Expression of Hsp27 also prevents the translocation of Daxx from the nucleus to the cytoplasm, which is induced upon expression of Ask1 or stimulation of Fas [160]. Nucleolar phosphoprotein B23.2 (NPM-ALK) has a constitutive tyrosine kinase activity responsible for its oncogenic property through activation of downstream effectors, such as phospholipase C gamma (PLCgamma) and type IA phosphoinositide 3-kinase. Furthermore, Src-kinases, particularly pp60 (c-src), associate with and are activated by NPM-ALK in various cancer cells, with tyrosine 418 of NPM-ALK required for association with Src-kinases [161]. Figure 7C shows that DJ-1 interacts with DAXX, and sequesters Daxx in the nucleus, preventing it from gaining access to the cytoplasm, and from binding to and activating its effector, kinase apoptosis signal regulating kinase-1. This prevents triggering the ensuing death pathway.

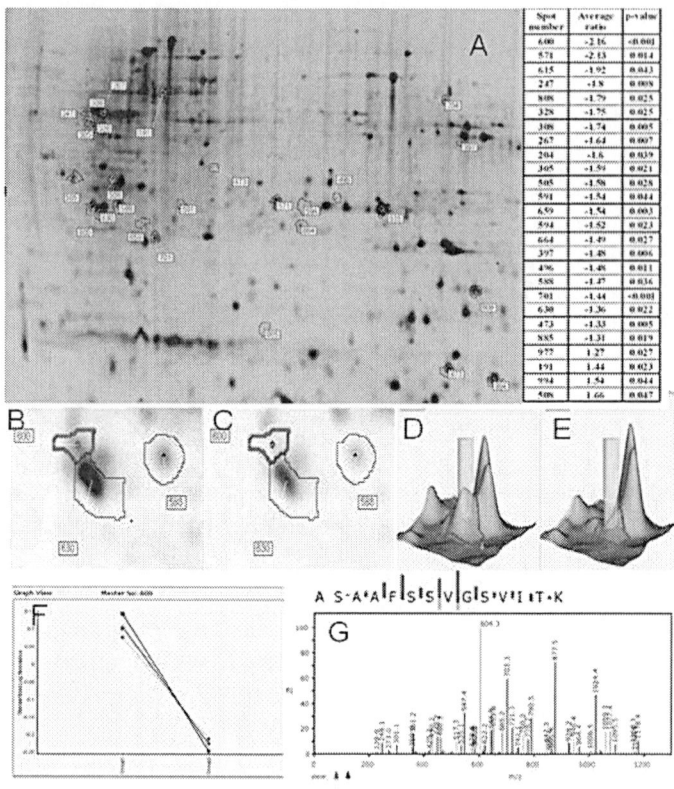

Figure 6. Proteomic analysis on the effect of f-PSA on PC-3M prostate cancer cells showing the differentially regulated proteins. (A) Representative SYPRO Ruby stained gel of f-PSA treayed PC-3M cells, PC-3M cells (2×10^5) were treated with10mM of-SA for48 hr, total protein was isolated, subjected to 2D-DIGE analysis and stained with SYPRO Ruby dye. The pH increases from left to right and the molecular mass decreases from the top to the bottom of the gel. Identified protein spots, differentially expressed in response to treatment with f-PSA, are outlined and numbered. Data represents an average of three independent experiments which yielded similar results. (B) Protein spot #600 from untreated control PC-3Mcells,.(C) Protein spot #600 from f-PSA treated PC-3M cells, (D) Abundance of protein spot #600 in untreated PC-3Mcells,(E) Abundance of protein spot #600 in f-PSA treated PC-3Mcells, (F) Graphical representation of statistical analysis of the control (Group1) and f-PSA treated (Group 2) groups for spot#600 by BVAmodule of Decyder software., (G) MS/MS analysis of the tryptic peptides obtained from protein spot #600 showing the unique spectra of tryptic peptide, ASAAFSSVGSVITK, which was subsequently identified as N8 gene product long isoform. X-axis represents the mass to charge ratio and the Y-axis represents the relative abundance. The mass range scanned was 0 -1500 amu.

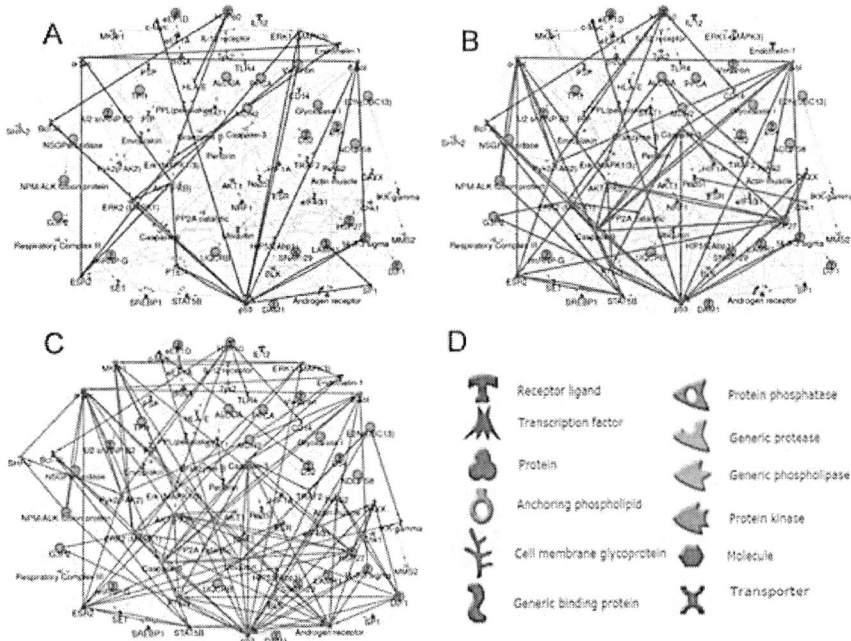

Figure 7. Involvement of identified proteins that are regulated in PC-3M by f-PSA treatment in biological pathways. Networks were generated by MetaCore analysis by combining relevant pathways involved in cancer pathogenesis. Differentially expressed proteins (circles) were mapped into the biological networks. (A) Networks involved in neoplastic events, (B) Networks involved in regulation of apoptosis and cell death, (C) A merged network of proteins involved in pathways including intracellular signaling cascade, cell differentiation and stress response. Highlighted lines represent the specific, designated pathways. Background lines represent secondary, related biological pathways; green and redlines represent activation and inhibition pathways respectively and (D) Various network legends used in the MetaCore mapping.

These findings suggest that the regulated sequestration of Daxx in the nucleus, keeping apoptosis signal-regulating kinase-1 activation in check, is a critical mechanism by which DJ-1 exerts its cytoprotective function [162]. To examine the relevance of the proteins/genes of prostate cancer cells whose expression was regulated by PSA with regard to cancer progression and metastasis, we searched the cancer profiling Oncomine database (www.oncomine.org) [163,164]. This database is a common repository for transcriptome meta-analysis of human cancers and tissues, and documents the genes whose expression is significantly modulated in cancer. An Oncomine search revealed that the majority of genes corresponding to proteins that were down-regulated by PSA in this study are elevated in various human cancers. Out of the 26 proteins identified as down-regulated by PSA, 13 were reported to be elevated in prostate cancer, and 5 were elevated in metastatic prostate cancer. Thus, the PSA-mediated down regulation of expression of proteins known to be elevated in prostate cancer, suggests that these proteins may contribute to the pathogenesis of prostate cancer and down-regulation of their expression may have a therapeutic benefit.

Conclusion

Demonstration that PSA sequestered in the tissue microenvironment has a major function as a regulator of angiogenesis could identify an important adjuvant therapy, or mono-therapy, for management of localized prostate cancer. Importantly, PSA replacement therapy would not generate an immune response. The natural loss of PSA with age, with progression of prostate cancer and/or as a consequence of androgen deprivation therapy could be reversed by introduction of PSA. Furthermore, published studies suggest that PSA may have important anti-angiogenic activity in other cancers, including breast cancer.

Table 2. List of proteins down-regulated in PC-3M cells in response to PSA treatment*

Spot No	Gene name	Accession Number	No of Peptides identified	Sequence coverage (%)	Calculated Mr (kDa)	Calculated pI	Molecular Functions
600	N 8 gene product long isoform	gi:1488414	2	13	26.4	6.13	Embryogenesis
571	Heat-shock protein beta-1 (Hsp27)	gi:19855073	9	32.2	22.7	6.4	Molecular chaperon Phosphoprotein, Stress response
571	Peroxiredoxin-6 (NSGPeroxidoxin)	gi:1718024	5	25.6	24.9	6.4	Edox regulation of the cell,.regulation of phospholipid turnover
615	Triosephosphate isomerase 1(TPI1)	gi:4507645	32	69	26.7		Triose-phosphate isomerase activity,Interconverting Aldoses and Ketoses;
247	Vimentin	gi:55977767	2	4.1	53.6	5.06	Structural molecule activity, cell motility, protein binding
808	Peptidylprolyl isomerase F (ppif)	gi:5031987	8	35	22.0		Accelerate the folding of proteins
328	Elongation factor 1-delta (eEF1D)	gi:20141357	1	5	30.9	5.0	Signal transducer activity, nucleic acid binding
308	Laminin receptor 1 (LAMR1)	gi:9845502	4	13	32.8	4.79	Cell adhesion,laminin receptor activity
267	Nucleolar phosphoprotein B23.2 (NPM/ALK)	gi:114763	3	11	28.4	4.5	RNA, nucleic acid, protein binding

Spot No	Gene name	Accession Number	No of Peptides identified	Sequence coverage (%)	Calculated Mr (kDa)	Calculated pI	Molecular Functions
204	Fructose-bisphosphate Aldolase A (ALDOA)	gi:113606	11	25.1	39.2	8.1	Lyase activity, catalytic activity
305	Nucleophosmin (NPM)	gi:114762	2	3.1	32.6	4.8	RNA, nucleic acid, protein binding
505	Heat shock protein 60 (HSP60)	gi:129379]	2	3.7	61.0	5.9	ATP binding, chaperone binding,
659	NADH dehydrogenase (NDUFS8)	gi:4505371	2	8.1	23.7	6.0	Electron carrier activity, oxidoreductase activity
591	BCAS2 protein homolog	gi:62899833	1	4.9	25.8	4.8	
591	U2 small nuclear ribonucleoprotein B (U2 snRNP B2)	gi:134095	2	8.4	25.4	9.7	RNA, nucleic acid, protein binding
594	Apoptosis inhibitor FKSG2	gi:20138343	1	4	20.3	5.1	Apoptosis
664	Protein DJ-1 (DJ1)	gi:56404943	3	13.8	19.8	6.8	Cell-growth promoting, transforming.
397	Glyceraldehyde-3-phosphate dehydrogenase(G3P2)	gi:7669492	2	8.7	36.0	8.57	Glycolytic activity, membrane trafficking, oxidoreductase activity
397	Malate dehydrogenase (MDH2)	gi:6648067	2	6.8	35.5	8.92	Oxidoreductase activity, lactate dehydrogenase activity
496	Cathepsin A (PPCA)	gi:20178316	2	3.8	54.4	6.6	Carboxypeptidase activity, peptidase activity
588	Lactoylglutathione lyase(Glyoxalase)	gi:134039205	2	4.9	20.6	5.5	Metal ion binding, lyase activity

Table 2. (Continued).

Spot No	Gene name	Accession Number	No of Peptides identified	Sequence coverage (%)	Calculated Mr (kDa)	Calculated pI	Molecular Functions
588	Tumor protein D52 (D52)	gi:1706289	1	6	19.9	5.0	Calcium ion binding, protein heterodimerization activity
701	ATP synthase H+ transporting (ATP5H)	gi:5453559	5	27	18.5	5.21	Hydrogen ion transporting ATP synthase activity
630	Stratifin (14-3-3 sigma)	gi:398953	2	6.9	27.8	4.7	Protein kinase C inhibitor activity, protein binding
473	Synaptosomal-associated protein 29 (SNAP-29)	gi:4759154	6	16	29.0	5.56	Transport, membrane fusion
885	Ubiquitin-conjugating enzyme E2 N(UCB13)	gi:46577660	2	13.8	17.1	6.6	Ligase activity, protein binding

*PC-3M cells were cultured with and without PSA (10μM) for 48 hr. Proteins were extracted and subjected to DIGE analysis. Data represents statistically significant down regulated proteins in response to PSA treatment (Student's t-test; n=3) that were identified using HPLC-MS/MS. Data is shown as protein name, gene accession number (Gi No.), number of peptides identified, % sequence coverage of the identified peptide, theoretical mass, pI and the known function(s) of the identified protein. Gene ID used in MetaCore analysis is given next to the each gene name.

Table 3. (Up-regulated proteins) PC-3M were cultured with and without PSA (10μM) for 48 hr (n = 3 independent experiments using 3 different PC-3M cultures). Protein was extracted and subjected to DIGE analysis. Data represent statistically significant differentially expressed (Up and down regulated) proteins with PSA treatment (Student's t-test) that were identified using HPLC-MS/MS. Data are represented as protein name, gene accession number (Gi No.), number of peptides identified, % sequence coverage of the identified peptide, theoretical mass and pI and the known functions of the identified protein

Spot No	Gene name	Accession Number	No of Peptides identified	Sequence coverage (%)	Calculated Mr (kDa)	Calculated pI	Molecular Functions
977	Human Platelet Profilin Complexed With The L-Pro10 Peptide	gi:3891601	7	54	14.8	8.47	metal ion binding
191	Heterogeneous nuclear ribonucleoprotein G	gi:23503093	2	4.6	42.3	10.06	RNA binding
191	Human Platelet Profilin	gi:3891601	3	27	14.8	8.47	RNA, nucleic acid and protein binding
994	Ubiquinol-cytochrome c reductase binding protein	gi:5454152	3	23	13.5	8.73	oxidoreductase activity
508	Tumor protein D54 (hD54)	gi:20141658	2	11	22.2	5.26	Cell proliferation, protein binding

Acknowledgements

The authors acknowledge supports from Alliance Foundation, Roswell Park Cancer Institute, Buffalo, NY (KCC), Margaret Duffy and Robert Cameron Troup Memorial Fund for Cancer Research of Kaleida Health Foundation (SAS) and grants from the National Institute of Health (1RO1AI08556901A, (SAS)) and CA77739-(GJS).

References

[1] Simard, J; Dumont, M; Soucy, P; Labrie, F. Perspective: prostate cancer susceptibility genes. *Endocrinology*, 2002, 143(6), 2029-2040.

[2] Clinton, SK; Giovannucci, E. Diet, nutrition, and prostate cancer. *Annu Rev Nutr*, 1998, 18, 413-440.

[3] Robbins, AS; Whittemore, AS; Van Den Eeden, SK. Race, prostate cancer survival, and membership in a large health maintenance organization. *J Natl Cancer Inst.*, 1998, 90(13), 986-990.

[4] Parkin, DM. Global cancer statistics in the year 2000. *Lancet Oncol*, 2001, 2(9), 533-543.

[5] Diamandis, EP. Prostate-specific antigen or human kallikrein 3? Recent developments. *Tumour Biol.*, 1998, 19(2), 65-67, discussion 67-68.

[6] Herrala, AM; Porvari, KS; Kyllonen, AP; Vihko, PT. Comparison of human prostate specific glandular kallikrein 2 and prostate specific antigen gene expression in prostate with gene amplification and overexpression of prostate specific glandular kallikrein 2 in tumor tissue. *Cancer*, 2001, 92(12), 2975-2984.

[7] Lintula, S; Stenman, J; Bjartell, A; Nordling, S; Stenman, UH. Relative concentrations of hK2/PSA mRNA in benign and malignant prostatic tissue. *Prostate*, 2005, 63(4), 324-329.

[8] Ahlgren, G; Rannevik, G; Lilja, H. Impaired secretory function of the prostate in men with oligo-asthenozoospermia. *J Androl*, 1995, 16(6), 491-498.

[9] Lilja, H; Oldbring, J; Rannevik, G; Laurell, CB. Seminal vesicle-secreted proteins and their reactions during gelation and liquefaction of human semen. *J Clin Invest*, 1987, 80(2), 281-285.

[10] Lilja, H. A kallikrein-like serine protease in prostatic fluid cleaves the predominant seminal vesicle protein. *J Clin Invest*, 1985, 76(5), 1899-1903.
[11] Clements J; Mukhtar A. Glandular kallikreins and prostate-specific antigen are expressed in the human endometrium. *J Clin Endocrinol Metab* 1994,78(6),1536-1539.
[12] Yu H; Diamandis EP. Measurement of serum prostate specific antigen levels in women and in prostatectomized men with an ultrasensitive immunoassay technique. *J Urol 1995*,153(3 Pt 2),1004-1008.
[13] Yu H; Diamandis EP. Prostate-specific antigen in milk of lactating women. *Clin Chem* 1995,41(1),54-58.
[14] Yu H; Diamandis EP; Sutherland DJ. Immunoreactive prostate-specific antigen levels in female and male breast tumors and its association with steroid hormone receptors and patient age. *Clin Biochem* 1994,27(2),75-79.
[15] Yu H; Levesque MA; Clark GM; Diamandis EP. Prognostic value of prostate-specific antigen for women with breast cancer: a large United States cohort study. *Clin Cancer Res* 1998,4(6),1489-1497.
[16] Levesque M; Hu H; D'Costa M; Diamandis EP. Prostate-specific antigen expression by various tumors. *J Clin Lab Anal* 1995,9(2),123-128.
[17] Kucera E; Kainz C; Tempfer C; Zeillinger R; Koelbl H; Sliutz G. Prostate specific antigen (PSA) in breast and ovarian cancer. *Anticancer Res* 1997,17(6D),4735-4737.
[18] Lundwall A; Clauss A; Olsson AY. Evolution of kallikrein-related peptidases in mammals and identification of a genetic locus encoding potential regulatory inhibitors. Biol Chem 2006,387(3),243-249.
[19] Olsson AY; Lilja H; Lundwall A. Taxon-specific evolution of glandular kallikrein genes and identification of a progenitor of prostate-specific antigen. *Genomics* 2004, 84(1),147-156.
[20] Cleutjens KB; van der Korput HA; van Eekelen CC; van Rooij HC; Faber PW; Trapman J. An androgen response element in a far upstream enhancer region is essential for high, androgen-regulated activity of the prostate-specific antigen promoter. *Mol Endocrinol* 1997, 11(2),148-161.
[21] Cleutjens KB; van Eekelen CC; van der Korput HA; Brinkmann AO; Trapman J. Two androgen response regions cooperate in steroid hormone regulated activity of the prostate-specific antigen promoter. *J Biol Chem* 1996, 271(11),6379-6388.

[22] Kollara A; Diamandis EP; Brown TJ. Secretion of endogenous kallikreins 2 and 3 by androgen receptor-transfected PC-3 prostate cancer cells. *J Steroid Biochem Mol Biol* 2003, 84(5),493-502.

[23] Yu H; Diamandis EP; Zarghami N; Grass L. Induction of prostate specific antigen production by steroids and tamoxifen in breast cancer cell lines. *Breast Cancer Res Treat* 1994, 32(3),291-300.

[24] Cleutjens CB; Steketee K; van Eekelen CC; van der Korput JA; Brinkmann AO; Trapman J. Both androgen receptor and glucocorticoid receptor are able to induce prostate-specific antigen expression, but differ in their growth-stimulating properties of LNCaP cells. Endocrinology 1997, 138(12),5293-5300.

[25] Zarghami N; Grass L; Diamandis EP. Steroid hormone regulation of prostate-specific antigen gene expression in breast cancer. *Br J Cancer* 1997, 75(4),579-588.

[26] Yu H; Diamandis EP; Monne M; Croce CM. Oral contraceptive-induced expression of prostate-specific antigen in the female breast. *J Biol Chem* 1995, 270(12),6615-6618.

[27] Wang C; Yeung F; Liu PC; Attar RM; Geng J; Chung LW; Gottardis M; Kao C. Identification of a novel transcription factor, GAGATA-binding protein, involved in androgen-mediated expression of prostate-specific antigen. *J Biol Chem,* 2003, 278(34),32423-32430.

[28] Oettgen P; Kas K; Dube A; Gu X; Grall F; Thamrongsak U; Akbarali Y; Finger E; Boltax J; Endress G; Munger K; Kunsch C; Libermann TA. Characterization of ESE-2, a novel ESE-1-related Ets transcription factor that is restricted to glandular epithelium and differentiated keratinocytes. *J Biol Chem.* 1999, 274(41),29439-29452.

[29] Oettgen P; Finger E; Sun Z; Akbarali Y; Thamrongsak U; Boltax J; Grall F; Dube A; Weiss A; Brown L; Quinn G; Kas K; Endress G; Kunsch C; Libermann TA. PDEF, a novel prostate epithelium-specific ets transcription factor, interacts with the androgen receptor and activates prostate-specific antigen gene expression. *J Biol Chem* 2000, 275(2),1216-1225.

[30] Ruizeveld de Winter JA; Janssen PJ; Sleddens HM; Verleun-Mooijman MC; Trapman J; Brinkmann AO; Santerse AB; Schroder FH; van der Kwast TH. Androgen receptor status in localized and locally progressive hormone refractory human prostate cancer. *Am J Pathol,* 1994, 144(4),735-746.

[31] Piironen T; Nurmi M; Irjala K; Heinonen O; Lilja H; Lovgren T; Pettersson K. Measurement of circulating forms of prostate-specific

antigen in whole blood immediately after venipuncture, implications for point-of-care testing. *Clin Chem* 2001, 47(4),703-711.

[32] Christensson A; Laurell CB; Lilja H. Enzymatic activity of prostate-specific antigen and its reactions with extracellular serine proteinase inhibitors. *Eur J Biochem*, 1990, 194(3),755-763.

[33] Niemela P; Lovgren J; Karp M; Lilja H; Pettersson K. Sensitive and specific enzymatic assay for the determination of precursor forms of prostate-specific antigen after an activation step. *Clin Chem* 2002, 48(8),1257-1264.

[34] Verhamme KM; Dieleman JP; Bleumink GS; van der Lei J; Sturkenboom MC; Artibani W; Begaud B; Berges R; Borkowski A; Chappel CR; Costello A; Dobronski P; Farmer RD; Jimenez Cruz F; Jonas U; MacRae K; Pientka L; Rutten FF; van Schayck CP; Speakman MJ; Tiellac P; Tubaro A; Vallencien G; Vela Navarrete R. Incidence and prevalence of lower urinary tract symptoms suggestive of benign prostatic hyperplasia in primary care--the Triumph project. *Eur Urol 2002*, 42(4),323-328.

[35] Morgan TO; Jacobsen SJ; McCarthy WF; Jacobson DJ; McLeod DG; Moul JW. Age-specific reference ranges for prostate-specific antigen in black men. N Engl J Med 1996, 335(5),304-310.

[36] Oesterling JE; Jacobsen SJ; Klee GG; Pettersson K; Piironen T; Abrahamsson PA; Stenman UH; Dowell B; Lovgren T; Lilja H. Free, complexed and total serum prostate specific antigen, the establishment of appropriate reference ranges for their concentrations and ratios. *J Urol* 1995, 154(3), 1090-1095.

[37] Borer JG; Sherman J; Solomon MC; Plawker MW; Macchia RJ. Age specific prostate specific antigen reference ranges, population specific. *J Urol* 1998, 159(2), 444-448.

[38] Stenman UH; Leinonen J; Zhang WM; Finne P. Prostate-specific antigen. *Semin Cancer Biol* 1999, 9(2), 83-93.

[39] Bindukumar B; Kawinski E; Cherrin C; Gambino LM; Nair MP; Schwartz SA; Chadha KC. Two step procedure for purification of enzymatically active prostate-specific antigen from seminal plasma. *J Chromatogr B Analyt Technol Biomed Life Sci,* 2004, 813(1-2), 113-120.

[40] Magklara A; Scorilas A; Stephan C; Kristiansen GO; Hauptmann S; Jung K, Diamandis EP. Decreased concentrations of prostate-specific antigen and human glandular kallikrein 2 in malignant versus nonmalignant prostatic tissue. *Urology*, 2000, 56(3),527-532.

[41] Stege RH; Tribukait B; Carlstrom KA; Grande M; Pousette AH. Tissue PSA from fine-needle biopsies of prostatic carcinoma as related to serum PSA, clinical stage, cytological grade, and DNA ploidy. *Prostate* 1999, 38(3),183-188.

[42] Grande M; Carlstrom K; Lundh Rozell B; Eneroth P; Stege R; Pousette A. Tissue concentrations of tissue polypeptide antigen (TPA) and prostatic specific antigen (PSA) in 42 patients with prostatic carcinoma. *Prostate,* 2000, 45(4),299-303.

[43] Qiu SD; Young CY; Bilhartz DL; Prescott JL; Farrow GM; He WW; Tindall DJ. In situ hybridization of prostate-specific antigen mRNA in human prostate. *J Urol*, 1990, 144(6),1550-1556.

[44] Pretlow TG; Pretlow TP; Yang B; Kaetzel CS; Delmoro CM; Kamis SM; Bodner DR; Kursh E; Resnick MI; Bradley EL; Jr. Tissue concentrations of prostate-specific antigen in prostatic carcinoma and benign prostatic hyperplasia. *Int J Cancer*, 1991, 49(5),645-649.

[45] Yu H; Diamandis EP; Levesque M; Giai M; Roagna R; Ponzone R; Sismondi P; Monne M; Croce CM. Prostate specific antigen in breast cancer, benign breast disease and normal breast tissue. *Breast Cancer Res Treat*, 1996, 40(2),171-178.

[46] Stege R; Grande M; Carlstrom K; Tribukait B; Pousette A. Prognostic significance of tissue prostate-specific antigen in endocrine-treated prostate carcinomas. *Clin Cancer Res*, 2000, 6(1), 160-165.

[47] Pousette A; Grande M; Carlstrom K; Stege R. Tissue PSA is the best predicting variable for the outcome of endocrine treatment of prostatic carcinoma. *Scand J Clin Lab Invest Suppl*, 1999, 229,27-32.

[48] Hasenson M; Lundh B; Stege R; Carlstrom K; Pousette A. PAP and PSA in prostatic carcinoma cell lines and aspiration biopsies, relation to hormone sensitivity and to cytological grading. *Prostate*, 1989, 14(2), 83-90.

[49] Ung JO; Richie JP; Chen MH; Renshaw AA; D'Amico AV. Evolution of the presentation and pathologic and biochemical outcomes after radical prostatectomy for patients with clinically localized prostate cancer diagnosed during the PSA era. *Urology*, 2002, 60(3), 458-463.

[50] Aus G; Damber JE; Khatami A; Lilja H; Stranne J; Hugosson J. Individualized screening interval for prostate cancer based on prostate-specific antigen level: results of a prospective, randomized, population-based study. *Arch Intern Med*, 2005, 165(16), 1857-1861.

[51] Gann PH; Hennekens CH; Stampfer MJ. A prospective evaluation of plasma prostate-specific antigen for detection of prostatic cancer. *Jama*, 1995, 273(4), 289-294.

[52] Stenman UH; Hakama M; Knekt P; Aromaa A; Teppo L; Leinonen J. Serum concentrations of prostate specific antigen and its complex with alpha 1-antichymotrypsin before diagnosis of prostate cancer. *Lancet* 1994, 344(8937), 1594-1598.

[53] Ulmert D; Serio AM; O'Brien MF; Becker C; Eastham JA; Scardino PT; Bjork T; Berglund G; Vickers AJ; Lilja H. Long-term prediction of prostate cancer: prostate-specific antigen (PSA) velocity is predictive but does not improve the predictive accuracy of a single PSA measurement 15 years or more before cancer diagnosis in a large, representative, unscreened population. *J Clin Oncol*, 2008, 26(6), 835-841.

[54] Andriole GL; Levin DL; Crawford ED; Gelmann EP; Pinsky PF; Chia D; Kramer BS; Reding D; Church TR; Grubb RL; Izmirlian G; Ragard LR; Clapp JD; Prorok PC; Gohagan JK. Prostate Cancer Screening in the Prostate, Lung, Colorectal and Ovarian (PLCO) Cancer Screening Trial: findings from the initial screening round of a randomized trial. *J Natl Cancer Inst*, 2005, 97(6), 433-438.

[55] Crawford ED; DeAntoni EP; Etzioni R; Schaefer VC; Olson RM; Ross CA. Serum prostate-specific antigen and digital rectal examination for early detection of prostate cancer in a national community-based program. The Prostate Cancer Education Council. *Urology*, 1996, 47(6), 863-869.

[56] Hugosson J; Aus G; Lilja H; Lodding P; Pihl CG. Results of a randomized, population-based study of biennial screening using serum prostate-specific antigen measurement to detect prostate carcinoma. *Cancer*, 2004, 100(7), 1397-1405.

[57] Thompson IM; Chi C; Ankerst DP; Goodman PJ; Tangen CM; Lippman SM; Lucia MS; Parnes HL; Coltman CA; Jr. Effect of finasteride on the sensitivity of PSA for detecting prostate cancer. *J Natl Cancer Inst*, 2006, 98(16), 1128-1133.

[58] Thompson IM; Pauler DK; Goodman PJ; Tangen CM; Lucia MS; Parnes HL; Minasian LM; Ford LG; Lippman SM; Crawford ED; Crowley JJ; Coltman CA; Jr. Prevalence of prostate cancer among men with a prostate-specific antigen level < or =4.0 ng per milliliter. *N Engl J Med*, 2004, 350(22), 2239-2246.

[59] Thompson IM; Ankerst DP; Chi C; Lucia MS; Goodman PJ; Crowley JJ; Parnes HL; Coltman CA; Jr. Operating characteristics of prostate-

specific antigen in men with an initial PSA level of 3.0 ng/ml or lower. *Jama*, 2005, 294(1), 66-70.

[60] Thompson IM; Ankerst DP; Chi C; Goodman PJ; Tangen CM; Lucia MS; Feng Z; Parnes HL; Coltman CA; Jr. Assessing prostate cancer risk: results from the Prostate Cancer Prevention Trial. *J Natl Cancer Inst*, 2006, 98(8), 529-534.

[61] Malonne H; Langer I; Kiss R; Atassi G. Mechanisms of tumor angiogenesis and therapeutic implications: angiogenesis inhibitors. Clin Exp Metastasis 1999,17(1),1-14.

[62] Desai SB; Libutti SK. Tumor angiogenesis and endothelial cell modulatory factors. *J Immunother*, 1999, 22(3), 186-211.

[63] van Hinsbergh VW; Collen A; Koolwijk P. Angiogenesis and anti-angiogenesis, perspectives for the treatment of solid tumors. *Ann Oncol*, 1999, 10 Suppl 4, 60-63.

[64] Liotta LA; Steeg PS; Stetler-Stevenson WG. Cancer metastasis and angiogenesis: an imbalance of positive and negative regulation. *Cell*, 1991, 64(2), 327-336.

[65] Folkman J. Angiogenesis in cancer, vascular, rheumatoid and other disease. *Nat Med*, 1995, 1(1), 27-31.

[66] Izawa JI; Dinney CP. The role of angiogenesis in prostate and other urologic cancers: a review. *Cmaj*, 2001, 164(5), 662-670.

[67] Wakui S; Furusato M; Itoh T; Sasaki H; Akiyama A; Kinoshita I; Asano K; Tokuda T; Aizawa S; Ushigome S. Tumour angiogenesis in prostatic carcinoma with and without bone marrow metastasis: a morphometric study. *J Pathol*, 1992, 168(3), 257-262.

[68] Furusato M; Wakui S; Sasaki H; Ito K; Ushigome S. Tumour angiogenesis in latent prostatic carcinoma. *Br J Cancer*, 1994, 70(6), 1244-1246.

[69] Folkman J; Klagsbrun M. Angiogenic factors. *Science*, 1987, 235(4787), 442-447.

[70] Folkman J. What is the evidence that tumors are angiogenesis dependent? *J Natl Cancer Inst*, 1990, 82(1), 4-6.

[71] Hanahan D; Folkman J. Patterns and emerging mechanisms of the angiogenic switch during tumorigenesis. *Cell*, 1996, 86(3), 353-364.

[72] Hori A; Sasada R; Matsutani E; Naito K; Sakura Y; Fujita T; Kozai Y. Suppression of solid tumor growth by immunoneutralizing monoclonal antibody against human basic fibroblast growth factor. *Cancer Res*, 1991, 51(22), 6180-6184.

[73] Aalinkeel R; Nair MP; Sufrin G; Mahajan SD; Chadha KC; Chawda RP; Schwartz SA. Gene expression of angiogenic factors correlates with metastatic potential of prostate cancer cells. *Cancer Res*, 2004, 64(15), 5311-5321.

[74] Duque JL; Loughlin KR; Adam RM; Kantoff PW; Zurakowski D; Freeman MR. Plasma levels of vascular endothelial growth factor are increased in patients with metastatic prostate cancer. *Urology*, 1999, 54(3), 523-527.

[75] Ferrer FA; Miller LJ; Andrawis RI; Kurtzman SH; Albertsen PC; Laudone VP; Kreutzer DL. Vascular endothelial growth factor (VEGF) expression in human prostate cancer, in situ and in vitro expression of VEGF by human prostate cancer cells. *J Urol*, 1997, 157(6), 2329-2333.

[76] Ferrara N; Davis-Smyth T. The biology of vascular endothelial growth factor. *Endocr Rev* 1997, 18(1), 4-25.

[77] Claffey KP; Robinson GS. Regulation of VEGF/VPF expression in tumor cells: consequences for tumor growth and metastasis. *Cancer Metastasis Rev*, 1996, 15(2), 165-176.

[78] Borgstrom P; Bourdon MA; Hillan KJ; Sriramarao P; Ferrara N. Neutralizing anti-vascular endothelial growth factor antibody completely inhibits angiogenesis and growth of human prostate carcinoma micro tumors in vivo. *Prostate*, 1998, 35(1), 1-10.

[79] Melnyk O; Zimmerman M; Kim KJ; Shuman M. Neutralizing anti-vascular endothelial growth factor antibody inhibits further growth of established prostate cancer and metastases in a pre-clinical model. *J Urol*, 1999, 161(3), 960-963.

[80] Masood R; Cai J; Tulpule A; Zheng T; Hamilton A; Sharma S; Espina BM; Smith DL; Gill PS. Interleukin 8 is an autocrine growth factor and a surrogate marker for Kaposi's sarcoma. *Clin Cancer Res*, 2001, 7(9), 2693-2702.

[81] Green AR; Green VL; White MC; Speirs V. Expression of cytokine messenger RNA in normal and neoplastic human breast tissue: identification of interleukin-8 as a potential regulatory factor in breast tumours. *Int J Cancer*, 1997, 72(6), 937-941.

[82] Slaton JW; Inoue K; Perrotte P; El-Naggar AK; Swanson DA; Fidler IJ; Dinney CP. Expression levels of genes that regulate metastasis and angiogenesis correlate with advanced pathological stage of renal cell carcinoma. *Am J Pathol*, 2001, 158(2), 735-743.

[83] Inoue K; Slaton JW; Eve BY; Kim SJ; Perrotte P; Balbay MD; Yano S; Bar-Eli M; Radinsky R; Pettaway CA; Dinney CP. Interleukin 8

expression regulates tumorigenicity and metastases in androgen-independent prostate cancer. *Clin Cancer Res*, 2000, 6(5), 2104-2119.

[84] Ren Y; Poon RT; Tsui HT; Chen WH; Li Z; Lau C; Yu WC; Fan ST. Interleukin-8 serum levels in patients with hepatocellular carcinoma: correlations with clinicopathological features and prognosis. *Clin Cancer Res*, 2003, 9(16 Pt 1), 5996-6001.

[85] Haraguchi M; Komuta K; Akashi A; Matsuzaki S; Furui J; Kanematsu T. Elevated IL-8 levels in the drainage vein of resectable Dukes' C colorectal cancer indicate high risk for developing hepatic metastasis. *Oncol Rep*, 2002, 9(1), 159-165.

[86] Kitadai Y; Haruma K; Sumii K; Yamamoto S; Ue T; Yokozaki H; Yasui W; Ohmoto Y; Kajiyama G; Fidler IJ; Tahara E. Expression of interleukin-8 correlates with vascularity in human gastric carcinomas. *Am J Pathol*, 1998, 152(1), 93-100.

[87] Davidson B; Goldberg I; Kopolovic J; Gotlieb WH; Givant-Horwitz V; Nesland JM; Berner A; Ben-Baruch G; Bryne M; Reich R. Expression of angiogenesis-related genes in ovarian carcinoma--a clinicopathologic study. *Clin Exp Metastasis*, 2000, 18(6), 501-507.

[88] Fujimoto J; Sakaguchi H; Aoki I; Tamaya T. Clinical implications of expression of interleukin 8 related to angiogenesis in uterine cervical cancers. *Cancer Res*, 2000, 60(10), 2632-2635.

[89] Fujimoto J; Aoki I; Khatun S; Toyoki H; Tamaya T. Clinical implications of expression of interleukin-8 related to myometrial invasion with angiogenesis in uterine endometrial cancers. *Ann Oncol*, 2002, 13(3), 430-434.

[90] Chen Z; Malhotra PS; Thomas GR; Ondrey FG; Duffey DC; Smith CW; Enamorado I; Yeh NT; Kroog GS; Rudy S; McCullagh L; Mousa S; Quezado M; Herscher LL; Van Waes C. Expression of proinflammatory and proangiogenic cytokines in patients with head and neck cancer. *Clin Cancer Res*, 1999, 5(6), 1369-1379.

[91] Yuan A; Yu CJ; Luh KT; Kuo SH; Lee YC; Yang PC. Aberrant p53 expression correlates with expression of vascular endothelial growth factor mRNA and interleukin-8 mRNA and neoangiogenesis in non-small-cell lung cancer. *J Clin Oncol*, 2002, 20(4), 900-910.

[92] Galffy G; Mohammed KA; Dowling PA; Nasreen N; Ward MJ; Antony VB. Interleukin 8, an autocrine growth factor for malignant mesothelioma. *Cancer Res*, 1999, 59(2), 367-371.

[93] Rossi D; Zlotnik A. The biology of chemokines and their receptors. *Annu Rev Immunol*, 2000, 18, 217-242.

[94] Miller LJ; Kurtzman SH; Wang Y; Anderson KH; Lindquist RR; Kreutzer DL. Expression of interleukin-8 receptors on tumor cells and vascular endothelial cells in human breast cancer tissue. *Anticancer Res*, 1998, 18(1A), 77-81.
[95] Wang JM; Deng X; Gong W; Su S. Chemokines and their role in tumor growth and metastasis. *J Immunol Methods*, 1998, 220(1-2), 1-17.
[96] Duan Z; Feller AJ; Penson RT; Chabner BA; Seiden MV. Discovery of differentially expressed genes associated with paclitaxel resistance using cDNA array technology: analysis of interleukin (IL) 6, IL-8, and monocyte chemotactic protein 1 in the paclitaxel-resistant phenotype. *Clin Cancer Res*, 1999, 5(11), 3445-3453.
[97] De Larco JE; Wuertz BR; Yee D; Rickert BL; Furcht LT. Atypical methylation of the interleukin-8 gene correlates strongly with the metastatic potential of breast carcinoma cells. *Proc Natl Acad Sci U S A*, 2003, 100(24), 13988-13993.
[98] Kim SJ; Uehara H; Karashima T; McCarty M; Shih N; Fidler IJ. Expression of interleukin-8 correlates with angiogenesis, tumorigenicity, and metastasis of human prostate cancer cells implanted orthotopically in nude mice. *Neoplasia*, 2001, 3(1), 33-42.
[99] Reiland J; Furcht LT; McCarthy JB. CXC-chemokines stimulate invasion and chemotaxis in prostate carcinoma cells through the CXCR2 receptor. *Prostate*, 1999, 41(2), 78-88.
[100] Veltri RW; Miller MC; Zhao G; Ng A; Marley GM; Wright GL; Jr., Vessella RL; Ralph D. Interleukin-8 serum levels in patients with benign prostatic hyperplasia and prostate cancer. *Urology*, 1999, 53(1), 139-147.
[101] McCarron SL; Edwards S; Evans PR; Gibbs R; Dearnaley DP; Dowe A; Southgate C; Easton DF; Eeles RA; Howell WM. Influence of cytokine gene polymorphisms on the development of prostate cancer. *Cancer Res*, 2002, 62(12), 3369-3372.
[102] Lee LF; Louie MC; Desai SJ; Yang J; Chen HW; Evans CP; Kung HJ. Interleukin-8 confers androgen-independent growth and migration of LNCaP: differential effects of tyrosine kinases Src and FAK. *Oncogene*, 2004, 23(12), 2197-2205.
[103] Mizukami Y; Jo WS; Duerr EM; Gala M; Li J; Zhang X; Zimmer MA; Iliopoulos O; Zukerberg LR; Kohgo Y; Lynch MP; Rueda BR; Chung DC. Induction of interleukin-8 preserves the angiogenic response in HIF-1alpha-deficient colon cancer cells. *Nat Med*, 2005, 11(9), 992-997.

[104] De Larco JE; Wuertz BR; Furcht LT. The potential role of neutrophils in promoting the metastatic phenotype of tumors releasing interleukin-8. *Clin Cancer Res*, 2004, 10(15), 4895-4900.

[105] Bendre MS; Margulies AG; Walser B; Akel NS; Bhattacharrya S; Skinner RA; Swain F; Ramani V; Mohammad KS; Wessner LL; Martinez A; Guise TA; Chirgwin JM; Gaddy D; Suva LJ. Tumor-derived interleukin-8 stimulates osteolysis independent of the receptor activator of nuclear factor-kappaB ligand pathway. *Cancer Res*, 2005, 65(23), 11001-11009.

[106] Massague J. The transforming growth factor-beta family. *Annu Rev Cell Biol*, 1990, 6, 597-641.

[107] Choi YH; Choi KC; Park YE. Relationship of transforming growth factor beta 1 to angiogenesis in gastric carcinoma. *J Korean Med Sci*, 1997, 12(5), 427-432.

[108] Albini A; Iwamoto Y; Kleinman HK; Martin GR; Aaronson SA; Kozlowski JM; McEwan RN. A rapid in vitro assay for quantitating the invasive potential of tumor cells. *Cancer Res*, 1987, 47(12), 3239-3245.

[109] Ikeda T; Lioubin MN; Marquardt H. Human transforming growth factor type beta 2, production by a prostatic adenocarcinoma cell line, purification, and initial characterization. *Biochemistry*, 1987, 26(9), 2406-2410.

[110] Steiner MS. Review of peptide growth factors in benign prostatic hyperplasia and urological malignancy. *J Urol*, 1995, 153(4), 1085-1096.

[111] Knabbe C; Klein H; Zugmaier G; Voigt KD. Hormonal regulation of transforming growth factor beta-2 expression in human prostate cancer. *J Steroid Biochem Mol Biol*, 1993, 47(1-6), 137-142.

[112] Merz VW; Miller GJ; Krebs T; Timme TL; Kadmon D; Park SH; Egawa S; Scardino PT; Thompson TC. Elevated transforming growth factor-beta 1 and beta 3 mRNA levels are associated with ras + myc-induced carcinomas in reconstituted mouse prostate: evidence for a paracrine role during progression. *Mol Endocrinol*, 1991, 5(4), 503-513.

[113] Balbay M; D; Juang P; Ilansa N;Williams S; McConkey D; Fidler IJ et al. Stable transfection of human prostate cancer cell line PC-3 with prostate-specific antigen induced apoptosis both in vivo and in vitro. *Proc Am Assoc Cancer Res* (abstr), 1999, 49, 225-228.

[114] Heidtmann HH; Nettelbeck DM; Mingels A; Jager R; Welker HG; Kontermann RE. Generation of angiostatin-like fragments from

plasminogen by prostate-specific antigen. *Br J Cancer*, 1999, 81(8), 1269-1273.

[115] Fortier AH; Holaday JW; Liang H; Dey C; Grella DK; Holland-Linn J; Vu H; Plum SM; Nelson BJ. Recombinant prostate specific antigen inhibits angiogenesis in vitro and in vivo. *Prostate*, 2003, 56(3), 212-219.

[116] Bindukumar B; Schwartz SA; Nair MP; Aalinkeel R; Kawinski E; Chadha KC. Prostate-specific antigen modulates the expression of genes involved in prostate tumor growth. *Neoplasia*, 2005, 7(3), 241-252.

[117] Mattsson JM; Valmu L; Laakkonen P; Stenman UH; Koistinen H. Structural characterization and anti-angiogenic properties of prostate-specific antigen isoforms in seminal fluid. *Prostate*, 2008, 68(9), 945-954.

[118] Fortier AH; Nelson BJ; Grella DK; Holaday JW. Antiangiogenic activity of prostate-specific antigen. *J Natl Cancer Inst*, 1999, 91(19), 1635-1640.

[119] Habeck LL; Belagaje RM; Becker GW; Hale JE; Churgay LM; Ulmer M; Yang XY; Shackelford KA; Richardson JM; Johnson MG; Mendelsohn LG. Expression, purification, and characterization of active recombinant prostate-specific antigen in Pichia pastoris (yeast). *Prostate,* 2001, 46(4), 298-306.

[120] Chadha KC; Kawinski E; Sulkowski E. Thiophilic interaction chromatography of prostate-specific antigen. *J Chromatogr B Biomed Sci Appl*, 2001, 754(2), 521-525.

[121] Kawinski E; Levine E; Chadha K. Thiophilic interaction chromatography facilitates detection of various molecular complexes of prostate-specific antigen in biological fluids. *Prostate,* 2002, 50(3), 145-153.

[122] Gallardo-Williams MT; Maronpot RR; Wine RN; Brunssen SH; Chapin RE. Inhibition of the enzymatic activity of prostate-specific antigen by boric acid and 3-nitrophenyl boronic acid. *Prostate*, 2003, 54(1), 44-49.

[123] Wang MC; Valenzuela LA; Murphy GP; Chu TM. A simplified purification procedure for human prostate antigen. *Oncology*, 1982, 39(1), 1-5.

[124] Zhang WM; Leinonen J; Kalkkinen N; Dowell B; Stenman UH. Purification and characterization of different molecular forms of prostate-specific antigen in human seminal fluid. *Clin Chem*, 1995, 41(11), 1567-1573.

[125] Graves HC; Kamarei M; Stamey TA. Identity of prostate specific antigen and the semen protein P30 purified by a rapid chromatography technique. *J Urol,* 1990, 144(6), 1510-1515.

[126] Wu JT; Lyons BW; Liu GH; Wu LL. Production of milligram concentrations of free prostate specific antigen (fPSA) from LNCaP cell culture: difference between fPSA from LNCaP cell and seminal plasma. *J Clin Lab Anal,* 1998, 12(1), 6-13.

[127] Yousef GM; Diamandis EP. The new human tissue kallikrein gene family: structure, function, and association to disease. *Endocr Rev,* 2001, 22(2), 184-204.

[128] Sensabaugh GF; Blake ET. Seminal plasma protein p30: simplified purification and evidence for identity with prostate specific antigen. *J Urol,* 1990, 144(6), 1523-1526.

[129] Lovgren J; Valtonen-Andre C; Marsal K; Lilja H; Lundwall A. Measurement of prostate-specific antigen and human glandular kallikrein 2 in different body fluids. *J Androl,* 1999, 20(3), 348-355.

[130] Deperthes D; Frenette G; Brillard-Bourdet M; Bourgeois L; Gauthier F; Tremblay RR; Dube JY. Potential involvement of kallikrein hK2 in the hydrolysis of the human seminal vesicle proteins after ejaculation. *J Androl,* 1996, 17(6), 659-665.

[131] Kurkela R; Herrala A; Henttu P; Nai H; Vihko P. Expression of active, secreted human prostate-specific antigen by recombinant baculovirus-infected insect cells on a pilot-scale. *Biotechnology* (N Y), 1995, 13(11), 1230-1234.

[132] Stenman U; Finne P; Zhang W; Leinonen J. Prostate-specific antigen and other prostate cancer markers. *Urology,* 2000, 56(6), 893-898.

[133] Bull JH; Ellison G; Patel A; Muir G; Walker M; Underwood M; Khan F; Paskins L. Identification of potential diagnostic markers of prostate cancer and prostatic intraepithelial neoplasia using cDNA microarray. *Br J Cancer,* 2001, 84(11), 1512-1519.

[134] Dhanasekaran SM; Barrette TR; Ghosh D; Shah R; Varambally S; Kurachi K; Pienta KJ; Rubin MA; Chinnaiyan AM. Delineation of prognostic biomarkers in prostate cancer. *Nature,* 2001, 412(6849), 822-826.

[135] Luo J; Duggan DJ; Chen Y; Sauvageot J; Ewing CM; Bittner ML; Trent JM; Isaacs WB. Human prostate cancer and benign prostatic hyperplasia, molecular dissection by gene expression profiling. *Cancer Res,* 2001, 61(12), 4683-4688.

[136] Bindukumar B; Schwartz SA; Nair MP; Aalinkeel R; Kawinski E; Chadha KC. Prostate-Specific Antigen Modulates the Expression of Genes Involved in Prostate Tumor Growth. *Neoplasia*, 2005, 7(5), 544.
[137] Print C; Valtola R; Evans A; Lessan K; Malik S; Smith S. Soluble factors from human endometrium promote angiogenesis and regulate the endothelial cell transcriptome. *Human reproduction* (Oxford, England), 2004, 19(10), 2356-2366.
[138] Delves GH; Stewart AB; Lwaleed BA; Cooper AJ. In vitro inhibition of angiogenesis by prostasomes. *Prostate cancer and prostatic diseases*, 2005, 8(2), 174-178.
[139] Sommers CL; Walker-Jones D; Heckford SE; Worland P; Valverius E; Clark R; McCormick F; Stampfer M; Abularach S; Gelmann EP. Vimentin rather than keratin expression in some hormone-independent breast cancer cell lines and in oncogene-transformed mammary epithelial cells. *Cancer Res,* 1989, 49(15), 4258-4263.
[140] Qi C; Zhu YT; Chang J; Yeldandi AV; Rao MS; Zhu YJ. Potentiation of estrogen receptor transcriptional activity by breast cancer amplified sequence 2. *Biochem Biophys Res Commun*, 2005, 328(2), 393-398.
[141] Huszar M; Halkin H; Herczeg E; Bubis J; Geiger B. Use of antibodies to intermediate filaments in the diagnosis of metastatic amelanotic malignant melanoma. *Hum Pathol,* 1983, 14(11), 1006-1008.
[142] Cappello F; Bellafiore M; Palma A; David S; Marciano V; Bartolotta T; Sciume C; Modica G; Farina F; Zummo G; Bucchieri F. 60KDa chaperonin (HSP60) is over-expressed during colorectal carcinogenesis. *Eur J Histochem*, 2003, 47(2), 105-110.
[143] Bindukumar B; Schwartz S; Aalinkeel R; Mahajan S; Lieberman A; Chadha K. Proteomic profiling of the effect of prostate-specific antigen on prostate cancer cells. *Prostate*, 2008, 68(14), 1531-1545.
[144] Waltregny D; de Leval L; Coppens L; Youssef E; de Leval J; Castronovo V. Detection of the 67-kD laminin receptor in prostate cancer biopsies as a predictor of recurrence after radical prostatectomy. *Eur Urol*, 2001, 40(5), 495-503.
[145] Tillman JE; Yuan J; Gu G; Fazli L; Ghosh R; Flynt AS; Gleave M; Rennie PS; Kasper S. DJ-1 binds androgen receptor directly and mediates its activity in hormonally treated prostate cancer cells. *Cancer Res*, 2007, 67(10), 4630-4637.
[146] Chen SL; Zhang XK; Halverson DO; Byeon MK; Schweinfest CW; Ferris DK; Bhat NK. Characterization of human N8 protein. *Oncogene*, 1997, 15(21), 2577-2588.

[147] Malinda KM; Kleinman HK. The laminins. *Int J Biochem Cell Biol,* 1996, 28(9), 957-959.
[148] Malinda KM; Nomizu M; Chung M; Delgado M; Kuratomi Y; Yamada Y; Kleinman HK; Ponce ML. Identification of laminin alpha1 and beta1 chain peptides active for endothelial cell adhesion, tube formation, and aortic sprouting. *Faseb J,* 1999, 13(1), 53-62.
[149] Aznavoorian S; Stracke ML; Krutzsch H; Schiffmann E; Liotta LA. Signal transduction for chemotaxis and haptotaxis by matrix molecules in tumor cells. *J Cell Biol,* 1990, 110(4), 1427-1438.
[150] Kibbey MC; Grant DS; Kleinman HK. Role of the SIKVAV site of laminin in promotion of angiogenesis and tumor growth: an in vivo Matrigel model. *J Natl Cancer Inst,* 1992, 84(21), 1633-1638.
[151] Menard S; Castronovo V; Tagliabue E; Sobel ME. New insights into the metastasis-associated 67 kD laminin receptor. *J Cell Biochem,* 1997, 67(2), 155-165.
[152] Pupa SM; Menard S; Forti S; Tagliabue E. New insights into the role of extracellular matrix during tumor onset and progression. *J Cell Physiol,* 2002, 192(3), 259-267.
[153] Reich R; Blumenthal M; Liscovitch M. Role of phospholipase D in laminin-induced production of gelatinase A (MMP-2) in metastatic cells. *Clin Exp Metastasis,* 1995, 13(2), 134-140.
[154] Nabeshima K; Inoue T; Shimao Y; Sameshima T. Matrix metalloproteinases in tumor invasion: role for cell migration. *Pathol Int,* 2002, 52(4), 255-264.
[155] Menard S; Tagliabue E; Colnaghi MI. The 67 kDa laminin receptor as a prognostic factor in human cancer. *Breast Cancer Res Treat,* 1998, 52(1-3), 137-145.
[156] Satoh K; Narumi K; Abe T; Sakai T; Kikuchi T; Tanaka M; Shimo-Oka T; Uchida M; Tezuka F; Isemura M; Nukiwa T. Diminution of 37-kDa laminin binding protein expression reduces tumour formation of murine lung cancer cells. *Br J Cancer,* 1999, 80(8), 1115-1122.
[157] Waltregny D; de Leval L; Menard S; de Leval J; Castronovo V. Independent prognostic value of the 67-kd laminin receptor in human prostate cancer. *J Natl Cancer Inst,* 1997, 89(16), 1224-1227.
[158] Shan YX; Liu TJ; Su HF; Samsamshariat A; Mestril R; Wang PH. Hsp10 and Hsp60 modulate Bcl-2 family and mitochondria apoptosis signaling induced by doxorubicin in cardiac muscle cells. *J Mol Cell Cardiol,* 2003, 35(9), 1135-1143.

[159] Chipuk JE; Bouchier-Hayes L; Kuwana T; Newmeyer DD; Green DR. PUMA couples the nuclear and cytoplasmic proapoptotic function of p53. *Science*, 2005, 309(5741), 1732-1735.

[160] Charette SJ; Landry J. The interaction of HSP27 with Daxx identifies a potential regulatory role of HSP27 in Fas-induced apoptosis. *Ann N Y Acad Sci*, 2000, 926, 126-131.

[161] Cussac D; Greenland C; Roche S; Bai RY; Duyster J; Morris SW; Delsol G; Allouche M; Payrastre B. Nucleophosmin-anaplastic lymphoma kinase of anaplastic large-cell lymphoma recruits, activates, and uses pp60c-src to mediate its mitogenicity. *Blood*, 2004, 103(4), 1464-1471.

[162] Junn E; Taniguchi H; Jeong BS; Zhao X; Ichijo H; Mouradian MM. Interaction of DJ-1 with Daxx inhibits apoptosis signal-regulating kinase 1 activity and cell death. *Proc Natl Acad Sci U S A*, 2005, 102(27), 9691-9696.

[163] Rhodes DR; Kalyana-Sundaram S; Mahavisno V; Barrette TR; Ghosh D; Chinnaiyan AM. Mining for regulatory programs in the cancer transcriptome. *Nat Genet*, 2005, 37(6), 579-583.

[164] Rhodes DR; Kalyana-Sundaram S; Mahavisno V; Varambally R; Yu J; Briggs BB; Barrette TR; Anstet MJ; Kincead-Beal C; Kulkarni P; Varambally S; Ghosh D; Chinnaiyan AM. Oncomine 3.0: genes, pathways, and networks in a collection of 18,000 cancer gene expression profiles. *Neoplasia*, 2007, 9(2), 166-180.

Index

A

access, 37
acid, 60
adenocarcinoma, 10, 59
adhesion, 9, 42, 63
adsorption, 24
African-American, 1
age, 5, 7, 10, 41, 50
algorithm, 36, 37
amino, 24
amino acid, 25
androgen, vii, 3, 10, 36, 37, 41, 50, 51, 57, 58, 62
androgens, 3
angiogenesis, vii, 1, 9, 13, 15, 19, 27, 31, 35, 41, 55, 56, 57, 58, 59, 60, 62, 63
angiogenic process, 9
anti-angiogenic agents, 30
antibody, 10, 20, 23, 56
antigen, vii, 49, 50, 51, 52, 53, 54, 55, 59, 60, 61, 62
apoptosis, 19, 31, 35, 36, 37, 39, 59, 63, 64
aspiration, 53
atherosclerosis, 9
ATP, 43, 44
attachment, vii, 32, 35

B

base, 54
basement membrane, 6, 35
benign, vii, 3, 5, 12, 13, 14, 49, 52, 53, 58, 59, 61
benign prostatic hyperplasia, 3, 12, 52, 53, 58, 59, 61
bias, 7
biochemistry, 1
biological activities, 35
biological fluids, 60
biological processes, 36
biomarkers, 36, 61
biopsy, 7
blood, 5, 7, 9, 52
blood vessels, 9
body fluid, 61
body mass index, 5
bone, 11, 55
bone marrow, 55
bone resorption, 11
boric acid, 60
breast cancer, vii, 3, 4, 6, 10, 41, 50, 51, 53, 58, 62
breast carcinoma, vii, 58
breast milk, vii, 3

C

cancer, vii, 1, 4, 5, 7, 9, 13, 14, 17, 27, 33, 37, 39, 41, 49, 54, 55, 56, 62, 63, 64
cancer cells, vii, 6, 11, 13, 15, 17, 33, 37, 56
cancer progression, vii, 6, 37, 39
CaP, vii, 1, 3, 7, 9, 10, 13, 15, 17, 27, 33
capillary, 9
carcinogenesis, 62
carcinoma, 10, 53, 55, 57, 59
cardiac muscle, 63
catalytic activity, 5, 43
CCR, 10
cDNA, 58, 61
cell culture, 61
cell death, 36, 39, 64
cell differentiation, 36, 37, 39
cell line, 4, 11, 13, 14, 16, 17, 27, 51, 53, 59, 62
cell lines, 4, 11, 13, 14, 16, 17, 27, 51, 53, 62
cervical cancer, 57
chemokines, 57, 58
chemotaxis, vii, 58, 63
chromatography, 19, 21, 23, 27, 60, 61
chromosome, 3
chymotrypsin, 3, 5
circulation, 5
cleavage, 24
clustering, 27, 36
colon, 58
colon cancer, 58
color, iv
colorectal cancer, 57
Congress, iv
consensus, 8
contamination, 25
contraceptives, 4
copyright, iv
correlation, 10
correlations, 57
culture, 12, 14, 16, 30, 31
CXC, 10, 58
cysteine, 10
cytochrome, 35, 45
cytokines, 10, 13, 57
cytometry, 12
cytoplasm, 37
cytosine, 11

D

damages, iv
database, 36, 39
deaths, 1
deprivation, 36, 41
detectable, 3, 4
detection, 5, 7, 17, 54, 60
diabetic retinopathy, 9
diagnostic markers, 61
digestion, 17, 31
disease progression, 6
diseases, 5, 62
DNA, 31, 53
DNA ploidy, 53
dogs, 4
down-regulation, vii, 34, 40
drainage, 57
dyes, 33

E

ejaculation, 61
electrophoresis, 16, 21, 24
ELISA, 12, 14, 16, 21, 24
encoding, 3, 50
endocrine, 53
endometrial carcinoma, 10
endothelial cells, 9, 30, 58
England, 62
environment, 33
enzymatic activity, 18, 20, 21, 24, 28, 60
enzyme, vii, 44
enzymes, 37
epithelial cells, 3, 5, 13, 14, 16, 62
epithelium, 4, 51
estrogen, 62
evidence, 7, 15, 55, 59, 61
evolution, 3, 50

extracellular matrix, 13, 35, 63

F

fibroblast growth factor, 13, 55
fibroblasts, 10
filtration, 24
fluid, vii, 3, 6, 50, 60
Ford, 54
formation, viii, 9, 13, 17, 30, 31, 63
fragments, 17, 31, 34, 59
France, 1
fusion, 44

G

gel, 3, 13, 16, 21, 23, 34, 38
gelatinase A, 63
gelation, 49
gene amplification, 49
gene expression, 3, 13, 14, 18, 27, 33, 49, 51, 61, 64
gene promoter, 11
genes, vii, 3, 13, 14, 16, 17, 27, 31, 36, 39, 49, 50, 56, 57, 58, 60, 64
genetic marker, 27
genetics, 6
glucocorticoid receptor, 4, 51
glycoproteins, 10, 35
glycosylation, 24
grades, 3
grading, 53
grants, 47
growth, 9, 13, 17, 28, 29, 31, 35, 43, 51, 56, 57, 58, 59
growth factor, 9, 13, 17, 28, 56, 57, 59
GTPases, 37
guanine, 11

H

haptotaxis, 63
head and neck cancer, 57
health, 49

heat shock protein, 35
hepatocellular carcinoma, 10, 57
heredity, 8
histochemistry, 4
homogeneity, 27
hormone, 50, 51, 53
host, 13
human, vii, 3, 10, 13, 17, 20, 23, 27, 35, 39, 49, 50, 51, 52, 53, 55, 56, 57, 58, 59, 60, 61, 62, 63
humoral immunity, 13
hybridization, 53
hydrolysis, 61

I

ICAM, 13, 15, 17
identification, 24, 34, 50, 56
identity, 61
IFN, 14, 17, 28
IL-8, 10, 12, 13, 15, 17, 57, 58
image, 30, 34
image analysis, 30
immune response, 41
immunoglobulins, 23
in vitro, vii, 11, 17, 31, 33, 56, 59, 60
in vivo, 11, 13, 28, 31, 56, 59, 60, 63
incidence, 1, 7
individuals, 6
inducer, 19
induction, 19, 35
inhibition, vii, 30, 32, 39, 62
inhibitor, 21, 23, 35, 43, 44
injections, 29
injury, iv
integrins, 9
interferon, 31
interferons, 10
interleukin-8, 56, 57, 58, 59
ion transport, 44
isolation, 19, 23
isoleucine, 24

Index

K

keratin, 62
keratinocytes, 51
kinase activity, 37

L

lactate dehydrogenase, 43
leaks, 5
ligand, 4, 59
liquid chromatography, 34
locus, 3, 50
lumen, 6
lung cancer, 10, 57, 63
Luo, 27, 61
lymphoma, 64

M

macrophages, 11
magnitude, 6, 11
majority, vii, 3, 4, 24, 39
malignancy, 1, 13, 59
malignant melanoma, 10, 62
malignant mesothelioma, 10, 57
malignant tumors, 6
mammals, 50
man, 7
management, vii, 41
mapping, 36, 39
mass, 34, 38, 44, 45
mass spectrometry, 34
matrix, 9, 13, 17, 24, 31, 35, 63
matrix metalloproteinase, 11, 35
matter, iv
measurement, 30, 54
measurements, 12
median, 5, 8
melanoma, 10
membership, 49
membranes, 24
messenger RNA, 56
meta-analysis, 39
metal ion, 45
metastasis, vii, 6, 10, 13, 14, 17, 19, 27, 31, 35, 39, 55, 56, 57, 58, 63
methodology, 33
methylation, 11, 58
mice, 3, 11, 18, 28, 29, 31, 58
migration, vii, 1, 7, 19, 32, 35, 58, 63
mitochondria, 63
MMP, 17, 35, 63
MMP-2, 35, 63
MMP-9, 17
molecular mass, 38
molecular weight, 24, 34
molecules, 9, 63
monoclonal antibody, 55
morphometric, 55
mortality, 1
MRI, 28, 29
mRNA, 10, 13, 15, 33, 49, 53, 57, 59

N

Na_2SO_4, 23
NADH, 43
national community, 54
neoangiogenesis, 57
neoplastic tissue, 10
neutrophils, 11, 59
NH_2, 10
nodes, 36, 37
normal distribution, 34
nucleic acid, 42, 43, 45
nucleus, 37, 39
nutrition, 49

O

osteoclastogenesis, 11
ovarian cancer, vii, 3, 50

P

p53, 36, 57, 64
paclitaxel, 58

Parnes, 54, 55
parotid, vii, 3
parotid gland, 3
participants, 7
pathogenesis, vii, 9, 17, 39, 40
pathways, 36, 37, 39, 64
PCR, 13, 14, 16, 27
peptidase, 43
peptide, 31, 34, 38, 44, 45, 59
peptides, 31, 34, 38, 44, 45, 63
permission, iv
pH, 20, 23, 38
phenotype, 10, 58, 59
phosphate, 11, 23, 42, 43
Physiological, 19
physiology, 1
placebo, 7
plasma proteins, 23
plasminogen, 17, 28, 31, 60
PM, 23
polarity, 6
polymorphism, 11
polymorphisms, 58
polypeptide, 53
population, 52, 53, 54
predictive accuracy, 54
preparation, iv, 25
principles, 19
probability, 8, 25
prognosis, vii, 6, 57
project, 52
proliferation, 9, 13, 19, 30, 45
promoter, 3, 11, 50
prostate cancer, vii, 3, 4, 5, 7, 11, 12, 13, 14, 16, 17, 19, 27, 31, 33, 36, 37, 38, 39, 41, 49, 51, 53, 54, 55, 56, 57, 58, 59, 61, 62, 63
prostate carcinoma, 53, 54, 56, 58
prostate gland, 6
prostate specific antigen, 49, 50, 51, 52, 54, 60, 61
prostatectomy, 53, 62
prostatitis, 5
protease inhibitors, 5, 20, 25
protein synthesis, 15

proteinase, 23, 52
protein-protein interactions, 33, 36
proteins, vii, 3, 17, 20, 23, 31, 33, 36, 38, 39, 42, 44, 45, 49, 61
proteolysis, 3, 33
proteome, 33, 36
proteomics, 33
PUMA, 64
purification, 23, 52, 59, 60, 61
purity, 19, 24
P-value, 36

R

race, 5, 8
reactions, 49, 52
reagents, 12
receptors, 9, 37, 50, 57, 58
recommendations, iv
recovery, 19, 23
recruiting, 11
recurrence, 62
recycling, 33
relevance, 1, 35, 39
renal cell carcinoma, vii, 3, 10, 56
reproduction, 62
residues, 10
resistance, 58
response, 3, 34, 36, 38, 39, 42, 44, 50, 58
rheumatoid arthritis, 9
rights, iv
risk, 7, 55, 57
risk factors, 8
RNA, 6, 13, 16, 42, 43, 45
root, 37

S

salt concentration, 23
secretion, 11
semen, 49, 61
seminal vesicle, 50, 61
sensitivity, 5, 7, 53, 54
sequencing, 24

serine, vii, 3, 20, 21, 23, 28, 50, 52
serum, vii, 1, 3, 5, 7, 11, 23, 30, 50, 52, 53, 54, 57, 58
services, iv
shock, 35, 42, 43
showing, 34, 38
signals, 9
silver, 21, 24
sodium, 20, 23
software, 34, 38
solid tumors, 10, 55
species, 4
sperm, 3
sprouting, 63
state, 6
states, 33
statistics, 49
steroids, 51
storage, 25
stress, 36, 37, 39
stromal cells, 10
structure, 24, 32, 61
structure formation, 32
substrate, 21, 24
sulfate, 20
Sun, 51
suppression, 13
survival, 6, 10, 49
survival rate, 6
susceptibility, 49
Sweden, 1
symptoms, 52
synthesis, 11

T

tamoxifen, 51
technology, 27, 33, 58
testing, 7, 52
TGF, 9, 13, 15, 17
therapy, viii, 36, 41
threshold level, 7
tissue, vii, 3, 4, 5, 13, 25, 31, 35, 41, 49, 52, 53, 56, 58, 61
TNF, 9

TPA, 53
trafficking, 43
transcription, 4, 14, 37, 51
transcription factors, 4, 37
transcripts, 10
transducer, 42
transduction, 63
transfection, 4, 59
transformation, 13
transforming growth factor, 9, 59
translation, 33
translocation, 37
transport, 6
treatment, 10, 17, 29, 34, 36, 38, 39, 42, 44, 45, 53, 55
trial, 7, 54
trypsin, 34
tumor, vii, 6, 9, 13, 16, 17, 19, 27, 28, 29, 35, 49, 55, 56, 58, 59, 60, 63
tumor cells, 10, 13, 16, 29, 56, 58, 59, 63
tumor growth, vii, 10, 13, 17, 19, 27, 29, 36, 55, 56, 58, 60, 63
tumor invasion, 13, 35, 63
tumor necrosis factor, 9
tumor progression, 19, 28, 35
tumorigenesis, 55
tumors, vii, 4, 6, 9, 28, 35, 36, 50, 55, 56, 59
tumours, 56
turnover, 42
tyrosine, 37, 58

U

United, 7, 50
United States, 7, 50
urinary tract, 52
urokinase, 28
USA, 23

V

variables, 10
variations, 6

vascular endothelial growth factor (VEGF), 9
vascularization, 11
vasculature, 9
VEGF expression, 10, 13
vein, 57
velocity, 54
venipuncture, 52
vesicle, 49
vessels, 9

W

wound healing, 9

X

X-axis, 38
xenografts, vii

Y

Y-axis, 38
yeast, 60
yield, 24

Z

zinc, 28